The
VIVA
Mayr
DIET

14 days to a flatter stomach and
a younger you

The
VIVA
Mayr
DIET

DR HARALD STOSSIER &
Helena Frith Powell

HARPER

HARPER

An imprint of
HarperCollins*Publishers*
77–85 Fulham Palace Road,
Hammersmith, London W6 8JB

www.harpercollins.co.uk

First published by HarperCollins*Publishers* 2009
This edition 2010

10 9 8 7 6 5 4 3 2 1

© Harald Stossier and Helena Frith Powell

Harald Stossier and Helena Frith Powell assert the moral right
to be identified as the authors of this work

A catalogue record of this book is available from the British Library

ISBN 978-0-00-730949-8

Find out more about HarperCollins and the environment at
www.harpercollins.co.uk/green

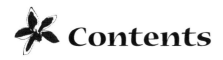

Contents

Acknowledgements

I would like to thank every single person who helped me realise this book. A special thank you to my wife Christine for her patience and medical support, to Carolyn Kohl for her PR enthusiasm and to Susanna Abbott and Charlie Viney for their confidence in this project. Finally, my special thanks go to Florian Klinger, the head chef at Viva Mayr, who devised the recipes in this book. His knowledge of good food and passion for flavour shine through his delicious dishes.

Dr Harald Stossier

EATING
Your
Way to a
HEALTHIER,
Thinner
YOU

Congratulations. This is the first step to a healthier, thinner, younger-looking and gorgeous you. I know what you're thinking: *All diet books say that.* Some of them even tell you that you'll get healthier and thinner just by picking up the book and paying for it. 'Buy this book, it will change your life,' they boast.

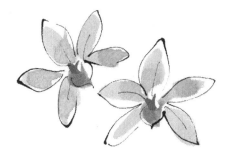

We all know they can't be telling the truth, but just as when we buy extortionately expensive face creams that claim to take years off our appearance, we want to believe them. We are desperate to believe that our lives can be changed – or, at least, that our hips can be slimmer – by reading a book, smearing on some cream or buying some new knickers.

The bad news is that most of the time it simply isn't that simple. There is no magic wand to make most of the changes that we want to see. But the good news is that the Viva Mayr Diet is as close as you can get to a miracle cure-all. It is, quite simply, the best diet there is – and the easiest one to follow. There is no calorie-counting, no weighing your food, and no living off cabbage soup for weeks on end. It is simply an approach to eating that will totally transform you. I guarantee that if you follow the Viva Mayr Diet, you will not only lose weight but you will also feel and look better than you have done in years.

This is because the Viva Mayr Diet is not only about what you eat, it is about how you eat and live. It is about making small changes to your everyday habits that will make a huge difference to your well-being. Some changes are so small you won't notice them. Others are more challenging. But once you have lived the diet for the 14 days outlined in this book, you will be converted, I promise.

Think about what you want to achieve. Why are you buying this book? You want to lose weight? You want to feel better?

To look better? Improve your health? I would guess that 99 per cent of you opted for losing weight as your number-one priority. Almost every woman I know thinks she should lose weight. But the fact is, as you will see from the Viva Mayr Diet, that weight loss is inextricably linked with all the other factors I mention. Like health and looks. One thing leads to another. Why not do it all at once and save time? Talk about multi-tasking …

Forget all fads; the raw-food diet, the blood-group diet, the 'whatever we haven't tried yet to convince people to part with their money' diet. Go for the Viva Mayr Diet, which is sustainable, logical, simple and extremely do-able.

Where to begin to be thin

So how to begin? This book is divided into 14 days, with one crucial Viva Mayr point of focus for each day. For example, the focus of Day Three is chewing, one of the most important elements of the Viva Mayr Diet. It's something we all obviously do – it's just that most of us don't do enough of it.

You can either read the whole book in one go and then go back and re-read the points on which you want to concentrate, or you can take it one day at a time for the 14 days, starting with the first chapter on getting prepared, and then progressing to when and how to eat. You'll also find all of the recipes you need for a new, thinner you at the back of the book, to help support you through your first 14 days and the beginning of your new lifestyle.

The Viva Mayr Diet is not over after 14 days; this programme simply gets you started. In reality, the Viva Mayr lifestyle is something you will want to carry on with for the rest of your life. Once you've changed the way you eat, you won't want to go back to your old habits. Viva Mayr is so different from other diets because it is about totally changing the way you think about food, and making food work for you to help your body reach its optimum state.

What is Viva Mayr?

Ironically, Viva Mayr hails from Austria, the country of Sacher-torte – possibly the most fattening cake ever invented. It all began with the Austrian physician Dr Franz Mayr (1875–1965), a medical legend. He was the first person to prove a direct link between digestive health and overall health and attractiveness. He developed the famous Mayr Cure, which thousands of people still follow to this day. Dr Harald Stossier, the man behind Viva Mayr, was head physician at the original Mayr Clinic for ten years before setting up on his own.

Dr Stossier is an extraordinary man. If he ran the world, there wouldn't be an overweight person in it. This is a man with a mission to change the world. Not through politics or good deeds, but by teaching us how to eat properly. Dr Stossier's theory is that to live a long, healthy and constantly slim life, all you need to do is make a few changes to the way you eat. He began his career as an electrical engineer, but after four years he understood his true vocation was elsewhere. At his wife's suggestion, he began to study medicine. However, early on he felt very strongly that traditional medicine was too narrow for him.

'I quickly realised I wasn't one of those typical medical students who just read the books and learned by rote. I felt very strongly my place belonged in complementary medicine,' he tells me, sitting at a table in the afternoon sunshine at the Viva Mayr Clinic on the shores of Lake Wörthersee in

Austria – the clinic he has created based upon his philosophy of health and well-being.

'When I left medical school I had the opportunity to work with Dr Erich Rauch, who had studied under Dr Mayr. Dr Rauch talked about intestinal cleansing as a real health issue. It seemed so perfectly logical to me and I quickly realised how important this message was for everyone.'

I'm not sure I'm ready to talk about intestinal cleansing with someone I hardly know, but apparently it is an issue that is paramount to good health. And a lot of people pay good money to come here to Austria and discuss it in great detail. Are they all slightly weird or should I let my inhibitions go?

Dr Stossier's clinic is an oasis of calm. Clients lie on sunloungers watching the boats go by and only need to get up for consultations with Dr Stossier, treatments or meals. It is not the most luxurious or the most expensive clinic in the world, yet while I was there I met several people who could well afford to go anywhere they chose. They have chosen Dr Stossier and his clinic in Austria because they believe that he can change their lives, and for the vast majority of people I met, he has.

I arrived at the Viva Mayr clinic one Thursday afternoon in August, starving hungry. I don't know what it is about clinics or diet places – or, indeed, just the thought of a diet – that makes me hungry. I can have just eaten Christmas lunch and start thinking about that diet I'm going to begin on New Year's Day and before I know what's going on, I find myself grabbing another roast potato to add to the 17 I've just eaten.

I shared a taxi from the airport with a lady called Brenda, from London. She had come to lose weight.

'I just need to stop eating,' she told me, as we sped through the Austrian countryside.

'Can't you do that in London?' I asked.

'No, I need to be forced to. I practically need a straitjacket and a cell. This is the only thing that works for me.'

'Well, if you get desperate, I've got some organic short-bread biscuits with me,' I smiled conspiratorially.

Brenda went pale. 'Please promise you won't give me any,' she pleaded, grabbing my hand.

I promised I wouldn't. Goody, all the more for me.

It was four o'clock when we arrived, and I was relieved to see from the timetable I was handed that dinner was at six o'clock. Not long to wait before I got some scoff. I said good-bye to my new friend and headed off to explore the place. My room overlooked the lake; it was a balmy afternoon, and there were people sunbathing. In the distance there was someone water-skiing.

The furniture in my room was modern and comfortable. There was a reclining chair that I could see myself becoming very familiar with, as I ploughed through all the books that Dr Stossier had given me to read as background research. I leafed through my welcome pack. Here I found a full of explanation of when and how to take Epsom salts (something about that made me feel rather nervous; aren't they a substance your grand-mother used to punish you with?), something called base pow-der, and a list of my various consultations. My first one was in half an hour, with the 'friendly werewolf' – as Dr Stossier has been called by various journalists because of his prominent mo-lars. I slipped into my bathrobe and flannel slippers in prepa-ration. Such a good look. Still, I was there for a reason, and I was going to embrace it.

The clinic is possibly the cleanest and most pristine place I have ever stayed in. It is on the shores of a beautiful lake in southern Austria. The rooms are all large with balconies, the staff super-smiley and friendly. Dr Stossier will not be drawn on the famous people who go there, but I get the impression from him and his wife, who also works there, that there are many.

'We have to respect their privacy,' he says. His wife is responsible for some of the treatments offered there, such as personality tests based on colours, and stomach massages. She is one of the warmest, most welcoming people you could ever hope to meet; she positively radiates good health and happiness.

If only we all lived the Viva Mayr way ...

I had first met Dr Stossier in London, at a meeting to discuss writing this book. The publisher had chosen me for the job because I have written two books in a similar vein – that is, with a mission to appeal predominantly to women. One was called *Two Lipsticks and a Lover*, which is all about how to get in touch with your inner Frenchwoman, and the other, *To Hell in High Heels*, is all about how not to age – from which staying thin, healthy, young and gorgeous is, of course, a natural progression. I also write a lot about beauty, health, women and diets in international magazines and newspapers, so I am a seasoned expert when it comes to knowing what works and what doesn't.

Dr Stossier and I bonded immediately in the canteen at HarperCollins HQ in London, where we discussed the central theme of the book. For years I have been convinced about the profound link between digestion and just about everything else – from how well we feel to how good our skin looks. I have suffered from digestive problems since I was a little girl, and have never really managed to cure them. In Dr Stossier and this project, I saw a way of finally understanding the whole process and changing the way I live to become thinner and healthier. I think he was happy to find a writer who was so in tune with the sorts of issues he has been working so hard to convey to people for so many years.

I first arrived at Viva Mayr with an open mind, ready to take everything on board. One of the great perks of my job is that I get to test everything for the reader. When I wrote my book about ageing, I travelled around the world testing anti-ageing techniques. At Viva Mayr, I was ready to test my own personal theory that if I started digesting properly, a whole myriad of problems, such as insomnia and bloating, would vanish. They did, and what was most incredible was the speed at which they vanished. What's more, I was not alone in being impressed with the results.

One man had been suffering from chronic diabetes for 15 years before he came to the clinic; since his first visit, he has suffered no symptoms at all. A lady I met had tried every weight-loss programme from Atkins to that well-known 'eat nothing until you are practically hospitalised' diet. The Viva Mayr method is the only thing that has worked for her. She had planned to stay for two weeks, and went on to book in for another three. In fact, everyone I met under Dr Stossier's care raved about his method and how good they looked and felt. These were people with a wide range of ailments, including obesity, diabetes and high blood pressure. But, according to the doctor, they all have one thing in common: irritated intestines. Dr Stossier estimates that around 90 per cent of us are wandering around with irritated intestines, which, if left to develop, can result in any number of chronic health conditions and diseases. In fact, he believes that almost every chronic illness we suffer from is related to problems in our intestines.

So how come everyone isn't hot-footing it over to Austria? Could it be that most people try to avoid thinking about their intestines too much?

'The reason people don't believe that diseases are caused by problems in our gut is that they live perfectly happily for, say, 20 years doing the same thing. And then suddenly they are taken ill with, say, diabetes. They assume this is something new but it's not; it's a slow process that has been building up for years and years, and which culminates in the disease, even though they seemed healthy before. If you look at a tree, for example, its health and strength does not come from its leaves; these are only a reflection of its health and strength. This comes from its roots, and you can't see if the roots are sick. Our intestines are our roots; they are not visible, but crucial to our health and strength. If they are weakened, so is the rest of the organism.'

Rather like a house that has a fault in its foundations, we go on for years thinking we're fine until one day we collapse. The point is you are not *either* healthy or unwell. The road from health to disease is long and full of small imbalances that do not yet constitute real illness. We don't often think about the impact of our behaviour on our health, or how we either undermine or support our natural desire to be healthy. Staying healthy requires a certain mind-set and a certain attitude, as well as a certain lifestyle. In practice this means having your own health in mind as a priority when you make all those small, everyday decisions.

Dr Stossier's theory is that we can avoid almost every disease and live a healthy, slim and happy life if we just learn to eat properly.

'We don't really think about eating,' he says. 'We just throw some food in and carry on with our busy lives. We have to re-learn this most basic human action.'

It is true that until I met Dr Stossier, I just ate. It didn't really matter to me *what* I ate, although I did avoid deep-fried Mars bars and other things that were guaranteed to make me fat. In fact, that was my one criterion for food – that it didn't make me fat. Apart from that, I didn't really care what I ate or when. And yet, I considered myself quite a healthy person. I exercised regularly, I didn't get drunk too often, I ate well (or so I thought) and I never drank caffeine. Surely that was enough to secure me a slot as a good person who looks after herself well? Apparently not.

There is something much more crucial than all of that put together, something that I had been neglecting: how I eat.

The right way to eat

To stay alive, we need to eat. Humans take in food, process it and then get rid of the end product. However sophisticated we are, the fact remains that the human species is part of a natural order. The types of food we eat and how we eat needs to reflect this. In other words, our eating habits need to reflect our biological roots and needs, and not just whatever happens to be convenient as we rush from home to work to the pub or the gym. There is a right way to eat and a wrong way, and, according to Dr Stossier, the vast majority of us are eating the wrong way.

Just what is the 'right way' to eat? There are endless books, arguments and theses on this subject. But the one thing we all agree on is that nutrition has a huge impact on our health and well-being. Most would agree that eating well plays a major part, if not *the* major part, in disease prevention. We were all told to eat our greens as children, and we all know why. Doctors are forever telling us to cut down on cholesterol and saturated fats. But Dr Stossier argues that it's not quite that simple. As well as eating those greens and avoiding saturated fats, you need to be aware of how and at what time of day to eat them, in order to help them to support your body to stay slim and healthy in the most effective way.

Nutrition influences our bodies in a number of ways. To live, we need a certain amount of energy, which we get from our food. We generally measure the type and quantity of food in the number of calories. But most people know from bitter experience that counting calories alone does not lead either to good health or even optimum weight. Whether we are calorie-counting or not, the vast majority of us manage to nourish ourselves more or less successfully throughout our lives. Most of us think that the majority of eating choices we make are good for us. Obviously we know when we're being 'naughty', but we let it pass and promise to be better tomorrow.

If we don't manage to be better tomorrow, we end up fat, and then go on a diet. I have read almost 100 diet books – not only in an effort to lose weight, but also to try and sort out digestive problems like IBS (irritable bowel syndrome), from which I am convinced I have suffered since childhood. I haven't found a single one that gave me a solution that was sustainable, logical and do-able.

What is missing from all the diet books I have read is logic, clearly defined guidelines and tangible results. In addition, I have yet to come across one diet book that is based on real medical and scientific knowledge. Most of them drone on about what to avoid, but they don't actually tell you how to optimise your health and lose weight at the same time. They just tell you about all the things you can't eat, which makes for pretty dull reading.

We all know that if we cut out dairy, sugar and wheat from our diets we lose weight. But is this actually good for our health, and how sustainable is it? How many times can you go out for lunch with your friends and eat nothing but a lettuce leaf before they stop asking you to join them? How many times have you struggled to lose weight by denying yourself just about everything you want to eat, only to put on every painfully lost pound within a few weeks? The Viva Mayr Diet is not about cutting things out of your diet and starving yourself. The Viva Mayr Diet is about changing the way you view food and eating, changing bad habits for good ones, thus ensuring weight loss and good health as well. Better still, it is also about ensuring that those pounds don't just pile back on again. It is a life-long way of eating, and if you follow the Viva Mayr philosophy, you will never be overweight again; it is simply physically impossible.

The Viva Mayr philosophy embraces good nutrition, and good nutrition is the best form of preventive healthcare there is. Luckily, we alone are responsible for our nutritional choices – put simply, we are responsible for what we put into our mouths. Good health is an ongoing daily aim and every day is the right day to start.

Taking responsibility

Health is created by our own actions and efforts, and we are solely responsible for it. Of course, accidents happen for which we cannot be blamed, but on an everyday level, you choose how well you're going to feel or how healthy you're going to be. You know, for example, that drinking 14 Tequila Slammers is not going to make you feel good. But it's your choice. Sometimes you just *need* those 14 Tequila Slammers (OK, maybe just a couple …).

The Greek philosopher Hippocrates noted that 'health arises when we actively seek it', and this premise is an important feature of the Viva Mayr philosophy, which defines the search for health as a positive thing. Health is quality of life in all its dimensions, which may vary from one individual to the next. We need to look at health as a natural and positive force that we each carry within us, and understand that it is within our own power to nurture. Quality of life as a parameter is attracting growing interest among scientists. There are even 'how to be happy' classes at Harvard University.

The word 'diet' comes from the ancient Greek term *diaita*. But, interestingly, this word didn't mean to the Greeks what it does today; rather, it meant 'way of life' or 'lifestyle'. In antiquity, living a health-conscious life was the obvious thing to do. This meant a disciplined approach to eating, including regular periods of fasting. Physical exercise and spirituality were also considered an important part of a healthy life. *Diaita* was far more than just a way to help people shed a few pounds, which is what the term 'diet' tends to mean now. This is also in keeping with the Viva Mayr approach to dieting. It is not a quick-fix to help you shed pounds (although it will do that), but an approach to adopt for life, to ensure that you not only stay thin, but also – more importantly – healthy.

Dr Mayr, the Austrian physician and Viva Mayr namesake, said: 'Nutrition is the result of the food we eat and our digestive system.' In other words, what matters is what we make of the food we eat.

When we eat a certain food – fish, meat, vegetable or potato – its nutrients do not go directly to the cells of our bodies. Our cells would not know how to make use of nutrients in this form. Instead, our digestive systems turn the food we eat into nutrients that our bodies can absorb and assimilate. Only then can we really make use of the energy and nutrients contained in food. Rather than saying 'you are what you eat', Dr Stossier and followers of Mayr would say 'you are what you digest'.

I am really excited about this book. It will provide the logic that I and so many others have been looking for, and explain the essential principles behind a thinner, healthier life. My aim is to take Dr Stossier's vast knowledge and expertise and present it to you in an easily digestible (pardon the pun) form of 14 main sections, set out as days of the plan. I will explain the reasons why it is so crucial that you overhaul your eating habits, and also how you can do so – easily and without too much pain, and for an enormous amount of gain.

Dr Stossier tells me that just by changing my eating habits I can put an end to my on-going digestive problems, lose weight, age better, feel better, sleep better, have more energy and clearer skin, concentrate on my work more effectively, and avoid major illnesses and disorders such as heart disease and asthma.

It seems a small price to pay for such a huge reward. I am keen to find out more.

The

FIRST
day of the
REST
of your
LIFE

You are about to discover:

How to prepare yourself practically and emotionally to begin the Viva Mayr Diet

How to make the famous Viva Mayr spelt bread

The shopping list you'll need to stock your cupboards with everything you'll need to get started

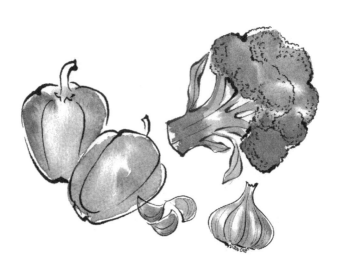

Today's Menu

Breakfast
Green tea, and fruit muesli with nuts (see page 230)

Lunch
Vegetable salad with chicken strips, and fresh berry cream
(see page 231)

Dinner
Soft polenta with steamed vegetables and herbs (see page 232)

This is the first day of the rest of your healthy, slim life. It's an exciting day. There are challenges ahead, but the rewards are huge. At the end of the 14 sections that comprise this book, you will be healthier and slimmer, and you will look and feel better. If you ever feel as though you can't go on, remember that these first few days are the toughest, but they are worth it. You are changing a lifetime of bad habits in order to hit your ideal weight, and also stay healthy and young-looking. That's a lot of reward, so of course there has to be some effort – even if it's minimal.

If you can, try to pick a weekend for the beginning of the diet, so you can prepare yourself and begin eating well on Saturday, and then launch into the body of the diet itself on Sunday.

So here is how you begin. You go shopping. Great start, eh? But sadly not for Louboutin shoes; rather, you'll be shopping for food that will enhance your health and keep you slim. During the 14 days that this book guides you through, you will be shown what to eat, how to eat it, when to eat it, and how to cook it. At the end of the book we provide recipes for every menu, designed to help you to take on board the focus of that section. So, for Day Three, which is all about chewing, you'll find a menu, with recipes at the back of the book, to encourage you to chew properly. Today we will look at the sorts of foods you need to stock up on to eat the Viva Mayr way. We will also be looking at how best to prepare yourself in other ways – such as mentally and physically.

If you're anything like me, the minute you know you're going on a diet you eat and drink everything you know you shouldn't. This is a mistake. Starting on a hangover is not a good idea. If you are hungover and tired, your body craves quick fixes like sugar and carbs to boost your energy levels, so starting a diet becomes doubly difficult. The ideal way to start would really be to fast the day before, so you would enjoy the taste and texture of all the healthy new foods. But I know this is not feasible for everyone, and fasting should never done without the supervision of a doctor. So give the fasting a miss and, for now, use this preparation day as a day to eat well (the recipes for today should be easy to make without too much extra shopping and effort), make the famous Viva Mayr spelt bread and think about the task ahead.

It's worth every ounce of effort

This is not something insignificant you have chosen to do. This is a huge undertaking that will transform the way you look and feel. I'd like you to think about exactly what it is you want to achieve and make a note of it. This would be my list:

- Lose weight.

- Sleep better.

- Have more energy.

- Look and feel better.

- Get rid of a pot belly and digestive complaints that have been plaguing me for years.

You can achieve this and more by sticking with me through these 14 days of the Viva Mayr cure. Remember that people pay thousands of pounds to go to the clinic – to learn all the things you are about to learn, and to eat the way you are going to eat for the next 14 days. What's more, you'll find that after your 14 days, your habits will have changed dramatically, and you'll be embracing a new way of eating, and a new way of thinking about what, when and how you eat. Viva Mayr is not a quick fix; this is permanent change we are talking about here. With this book, you have the opportunity to acquire all this knowledge and all those secrets for a fraction of the price and in the comfort of your own home. This is a great opportunity, and one I think you will be really happy that you took.

Make that list and keep it somewhere safe; look at it now and again to remind yourself why you are doing this. I promise that the rewards are huge compared with the actual effort. The Viva Mayr Diet is all about making subtle changes in your lifestyle that will result in huge gains both in terms of weight loss and your general health. This is something you need to keep in mind at all times. You have to be a little like a child waiting for Christmas; just a few more days and you'll see some results, another week and you'll have lost another few kilos. But when Christmas Day comes, you will be so hooked and happy with the new you that you won't want to stop.

As I said, there will be challenges. If you are a coffee and tea addict, you may get headaches as your body purges itself of toxins. I know this might sound silly, but look upon those headaches as a good sign. Headaches equal progress. A lot of people I met at the clinic said that the toughest day is Day Three, when you are really starting to feel the effects of what is effectively a deep cleanse. You feel headachy, tired and perhaps a little depressed, too. But then you come out the other side feeling incredible. Whatever side-effects you experience, they can never be as bad as feeling fat and unhealthy. So persevere and you will make it, I promise.

Re-read your list of aims, remind yourself why you are here and what you are doing. Remember that you bought this book with an aim in mind and a goal to reach – and you *will reach that goal*. There is no one stopping you. You have it within your grasp to become whatever you want.

Stocking up

So how best to prepare for the Viva Mayr journey? Today is not only a day to stock up on all the good things you are going to feed your new-look body, but also a great opportunity to throw out all those crisps and Mars bar ice-creams you have been saving for a special treat. You are going to prepare yourself both mentally and practically.

Your essential shopping list
Over the next 14 days, you'll need the following foods in your

store cupboard and fridge. Most of the recipes on pages 230–81 are designed to serve about four, so if you are cooking for your family, this is probably ideal; however, if you are going solo, you will need to purchase smaller quantities of the ingredients. Read through the recipes before heading off to the shops, so you know what you'll need. It's also a good idea to purchase your fresh fruit, vegetables and herbs daily (if possible), and, unless you have a very good deep-freezer, your meat and fish, as well.

Drinks
Green tea
Pomegranate juice
Spring water

Store cupboard
Stevia
Vegetable stock cubes, organic
Rock salt
Extra-virgin olive oil
Cold-pressed linseed oil
Cold-pressed hemp oil
Cold-pressed walnut oil
Cold-pressed pumpkin-seed oil
Coconut oil
Truffle oil (optional)
Balsamic vinegar
Honey
Maple syrup
Cider vinegar
Blackcurrant purée
Baking powder

Cream of tartar
Organic soya sauce
Raisins or sultanas
Green olives
Black olives
Dried fruit, such as apricots and prunes

Dairy & eggs
Organic eggs
Butter
Soft goat's cheese
Soft sheep's cheese
Sour cream
Soya milk
Single cream
Double cream
Parmesan cheese
Cottage cheese
Rice milk
Oat milk

Live sheep's, goat's or cow's milk yoghurt *(avoid the latter if you have any allergies or intolerance to milk, milk proteins or lactose)*

Goat's milk or sheep's milk *(full-fat cow's milk is OK, if you have no allergies)*

Fruit & vegetables

Apples

Berries *(such as strawberries, raspberries, blackberries, blueberries; whatever you can get)*

Pomegranates

Oranges

Lemons

Limes

Bananas

Papaya

Mangoes

Spinach

Onions

Radishes

Celery

Carrots

Fennel

Potatoes

Kohlrabi

Ripe vine tomatoes

Baby plum tomatoes

Pumpkin or butternut squash

Salad *(various lettuce leaves; anything goes)*

Garden cress

Mixed sprouts, such as fenu greek, alfalfa, mung bean, radish, soya

Courgettes

Parsnips

Avocados

Artichokes (globe)

Broccoli

Celeriac

Rocket

Aubergines

Turnip

Shallots

Fresh beetroot

Fresh horseradish (*or shop-bought horseradish sauce*)

As well as any fruits and vegetables in season …

Fish & meat and meat substitutes

Trout fillets

Smoked trout fillets

Skinless, boneless turkey breasts

Slices of turkey ham

Loin of lamb

Salmon fillets

Slices of smoked salmon

Fillet of beef

Organic silken tofu (or hemp tofu if you can get it)

Char caviar

Grains, pulses, nuts and seeds

Walnuts

Pumpkin seeds

Almonds

Whole linseeds

Chickpeas (dried)

Sesame seeds

Amaranth seeds

Ground oats

Buckwheat flour

Millet

Corn flakes

Spelt flour

Rice flakes

Soya flour

Polenta

Potato flour (an Italian deli should sell this)

Risotto rice

Herbs & spices

Note: some of the dried herbs can be found at your local health-food shop

Fresh ginger

Fresh lemon verbena

Fresh dill

Fresh chervil

Fresh tarragon

Fresh lovage

Fresh coriander

Fresh thyme

Fresh rosemary stalks

Fresh marjoram

Fresh mint

Fresh parsley

Fresh or dried fennel

Fresh lemongrass

Fresh basil

Cinnamon sticks

Ground cloves

Ground ginger

Ground cinnamon

Nutmeg

Vermouth

Dried caraway seeds

Dried yarrow

Dried horsetail

Dried birch leaves

You may also want to consider getting some crystals to energise and purify your water; rose quartz is a great choice, if you can get it.

So no doughnuts and no deep-fried Mars bars – funny that. If the list looks sadly lacking in sugar hits, just remember that your taste buds will change in a few days and you will no longer crave all those sweet things. You are perfectly capable of living without them, and you will start to feel and look better very quickly as a result of eating the kinds of foods listed above, which actually have some nutritional value.

Going off-piste?

It's perfectly acceptable to create your own meals rather than following the suggested menu plans, although you may want to try them for a few days first, to get the hang of the way food is prepared at Viva Mayr. On page 229, you'll find hints for cooking the Viva Mayr way, and a little later in this section you'll find out what foods you need, and why you should be eating them. By all means experiment with the foods listed above, or choose some of your own. The key words are fresh, organic (if possible), varied and whole. So get plenty of different whole grains, fresh, brightly coloured fruits and vegetables, a little fresh, lean meat and fish, some good-quality seeds and nuts, plenty of fresh herbs, organic eggs and some dairy – sheep and goat's, if you can; otherwise, cow's milk dairy produce will be fine, too. The most important things you can and should purchase are cold-pressed oils, which feature every single day on the Viva Mayr Diet (see page 43–46).

What about sugar?

When I ask Dr Stossier what type of sugar is best for us to eat, he is very firm when he responds.

'No sugar – that's the best sugar you can have.'

But that's totally and utterly impossible. How can anyone possibly live without sugar? I mean, even if you wanted to, how could you avoid it? Is there such a thing as sugar-free shortbread biscuits?

'I know it's difficult,' he concedes, 'but the fact is that you don't need any more sugar than you get from the food you already eat. We get so many different forms of carbohydrates that it is not necessary to add more.'

I ask him if brown sugar is better. Apparently it is not. How irritating is that? I have spent the last 20 years taking brown sugar lumps instead of white ones because I think they are healthier. I don't even have any white sugar in the house; I do everything with brown sugar, even baking – which is not easy if you're trying to bake a white fluffy sponge.

'Brown sugar is very often only white sugar that has been coloured brown to give it the appearance of natural, healthy sugar,' explains the doctor. 'In fact, natural sugar wouldn't even taste like sugar. If you have a sweet tooth then use the plant Stevia instead.'

I have tried Stevia in its raw form and also in a chocolate mousse. It is delicious and sweet enough for anyone. You can buy it online or in health-food shops. But be aware that a craving for sweet things is a sign that your cells are asking for sugar because they need energy to digest your food. This means you have not given your body the best chance to digest, and is not good news. You are either eating the wrong thing at the wrong time, not chewing enough (see page 55), eating too much protein (see pages 47–48) or eating when you are stressed (see page 167).

Fruit is a better option than sugar. Instead of sugar, sprinkle fruit on your cereal. An ideal breakfast would be muesli and some fruit followed by eggs (preferably not fried, sadly, which will upset my daughter who likes nothing better than to start the day with one or even two fried eggs), and some raw vegetables. While I was at the Viva Mayr Clinic, I had an avocado with linseed oil for breakfast – surprisingly delicious and one of the most nutritious ways to start the day. But if you can't imagine going on without your daily fix of doughnuts, Mars bars or fizzy drinks, please do me a favour and just give it three days; that's all it will take to break your nasty habits, for your taste buds to mellow, and for those things to seem like sugary, unhealthy and fattening blasts from the past.

Roll up your sleeves ...

Once you have all your ingredients stashed away, then it's time to make spelt bread. Spelt bread is one of the things for which the Viva Mayr Clinic is famous – or even infamous! Everyone who goes there, from film stars and property magnates to professional football players is put on a diet that includes spelt bread.

The first time you eat it, you may well be horrified. The bread tastes, well, stale. I can imagine the great and the good who visit the clinic – and are used to the better things in life – being rather shocked when they are presented with a bowl of vegetable broth and some, um, *stale* bread. But the point is that it teaches us to chew properly. Actually, I grew rather fond of the taste while I was at the clinic. Freshly baked, it is delicious, once you have learned how to chew properly.

Spelt bread is easy to make. You will need to prepare it the day before you want to eat it. I find it easiest to do the first part of the preparation when I get up in the morning and the second part when I get home from work. Here is the recipe:

Spelt bread

Makes about 15 pieces

Ingredients for the sourdough
Part one
125g sheep's or goat's milk yoghurt
125ml water
125g spelt flour

Mix all the ingredients together using a food mixer and leave to stand for 8 hours in a warm place (an airing cupboard is a good choice, or above an oven that has been previously heated). The dough is quite liquid at first but it will firm up as it stands.

Part two
750g spelt flour
250ml warm water
1½ tablespoons cream of tartar
½ teaspoon rock or sea salt
½ teaspoon ground coriander
½ teaspoon ground cumin
½ teaspoon ground aniseed
½ teaspoon ground fennel seeds
Sourdough (see above)

Mix all of the ingredients together with the sourdough and stir for 8 to 10 minutes. You might find it easier to use a food processor, or a mixer with a dough hook, rather than mixing by hand. The dough should be quite firm now.

Form flatbreads of approximately 70g each from the spelt dough. They must be very flat. Leave them to rise on a lightly floured baking tray for approximately 45 minutes, then prick and bake in the preheated oven at 190°C (375°F/Gas mark 5) for approximately 15 minutes. The breads should be golden brown and firm to the touch.

Leave them to rest for a day. That way they'll be a little harder. You can also freeze the bread until you need it. It will last for several days; in fact, Dr S encourages you to eat it after a day or two so that it is tougher to chew.

No time for baking?

If you don't have time, simply buy a packet of Ryvita, a rye or whole-meal loaf from the supermarket, or pick up some spelt bread at your local health-food store. I'd really recommend this recipe, though, as taste-wise it beats any bread you can buy hands down. Please do make the time today – in between reading – to make your first batch of spelt bread. You also need to make it well in advance because when it comes to learning how to chew properly, the bread should be a day or two old.

Cooking the Viva Mayr way

Once you know what to eat, how are you meant to cook it? The goal of cooking the Viva Mayr way is to create a dish that tastes good, while at the same time preserving the food's nutrients. Some methods are better than others because they make foods easier to digest. In many cases, food preparation is essential for us to be able to digest a food at all. Have you ever tried eating raw dried pasta?

By far the best way to cook vegetables is to steam them, and the best way to cook meat is to grill it. Fish can be poached, steamed or grilled. If you do end up frying, use only warm-pressed oils. Palm oil and coconut oil are especially suitable, because they have a very high smoke point of between 160°C and 180°C (320°F and 350°F), which means they can be heated without destroying the valuable nutrients. Heating cold-pressed oils turns them into trans fats – the very worst type of fats you can eat. If you do choose to cook with olive oil, or vegetable or seed oils, choose warm-pressed varieties. The fatty acids they contain will not be altered by cooking.

Contrary to what most other diet books will tell you, butter is fine. Butter contains milk fat, which has high levels of essential fatty acids, required for the brain and immune system. But don't heat butter. At the most, butter can be melted gently and used to coat vegetables. Heating any more than this destroys butter and robs it of its health benefits, by destroying the healthy fatty acid chains.

Dr Stossier suggests we all cook using more herbs. They are excellent for supporting the digestive system, they taste great, and they can add flavour to just about anything you eat. Think about using herbs in a more Mediterranean way. For example, use fresh mint in a salad, as you would in Greece, or make fresh pesto sauce with basil. Basil is extremely versatile and perks most things up; add it to some steamed vegetables with some olive oil to finish off, and suddenly you have a tasty and nutritious meal. Any boring salad can be spiced up with a bit of coriander. Next time you eat salmon, pop some dill on top.

In terms of equipment, the only kitchen appliance in which you need to invest is a steamer. If you're not yet convinced about the benefits of steaming food, just use a colander over a saucepan. But bear in mind that steaming preserves essential nutrients in food, such as the antioxidants, flavonoids, vitamins and minerals in vegetables.

You will also need a food processor or mixer for some of the recipes; if you don't have one and don't want to buy one, then do what your great-grandmother would have done and use a fork – and some wrist power!

What *not* to eat

So what foods should we avoid? Dr Stossier is pragmatic.

'I can't say this is best or this is better than others; we need them all. Each food has a different ingredient that our bodies crave,' he says.

I ask Dr Stossier if he would ever eat a doughnut. 'Not if there are other options,' he smiles.

'What about dark chocolate?' I ask him hopefully, 'and red wine – they're full of antioxidants aren't they?'

Dr Stossier looks at me with a wry smile. 'You would be drunk before you were able to reap any of the antioxidant benefits of red wine,' he says. 'Which would then of course outweigh any benefits. As for dark chocolate, if you want to enjoy a piece of dark chocolate now and again, then go ahead. But don't kid yourself that it is full of antioxidants.'

Prepare yourself emotionally

So are you ready for Viva Mayr? This has been a day of preparation for the new you. In terms of physical preparation it is fairly simple. You need to buy the food on the list (without succumbing to any doughnuts or bottles of beer) and also invest in a steamer if you can. You are easing into the diet with recipes made up from food you are likely to have at home. Begin and end the day with a cup of hot water with a slice of lemon in it.

Although we have not been through them all yet, there are some Viva Mayr rules you will need to follow today and from now on. They are:

- Chew as much as you possibly can.

- Eat nothing raw after four.

- Take at least 15 minutes of exercise a day.

- Eat more early on in the day, reducing portions in the evening.

Take some time for yourself on Day One. I have three children and know how difficult that can be. It is important that you have a chance to prepare both mentally and physically. Having said that, the Viva Mayr, unlike other diets, has an easy-to-follow menu that can be served to the whole family. There is no need to cook separately for anyone.

This is not a difficult diet in terms of what you eat, and you most certainly won't be horribly hungry, so throw yourself right into it. There are a few adjustments to your routine that will have to be made, such as eating a big breakfast and having dinner earlier in the evening. Start this diet with an open mind, and for 14 days I'll guide you through the ins and outs of the optimum way to eat.

Once you have been shopping, have a quiet night and end the evening with a cup of hot water, or herbal tea such as lemon balm, chamomile, or St John's wort. If you wish, add a slice of lemon. You need to begin to cleanse your system in preparation for the new you. Tomorrow is a big day.

In summary ...

- Preparing yourself emotionally, physically and practically will help to ensure your Viva Mayr experience is a success.

- Spelt bread is an essential on the diet, and making it can be a therapeutic experience, not to mention great practice for chewing properly.

- Make sure you have all the right foods at your fingertips as this will help to get you through periods where you run out of steam.

Case Study

Sally, 49, London

I have four boys, and have basically been overweight since the birth of the first one. Then things just got worse. I have been on more crazy diets than you can imagine. One involved nothing but celery (the idea being that you use more calories chewing it than you consume), and another involved eating nothing but boiled eggs and grapefruit. I was starving hungry all the time, and had to cook scrummy food like macaroni cheese for the children, which just added to my misery. As soon as I heard about Viva Mayr I thought I would try it because it sounded more realistic than anything else I had tried. I also realised there was no need to torture myself with cooking for the children, because they could just eat what I did and so could my husband.

I started on a weekend. The children and I made the spelt bread, and we stocked up on all the food. Actually, it was a bit of an adventure – a challenge – and we all got into it. They didn't like the spelt bread, but I did. I also tried to get them all to chew slowly, which with four boys was not easy. I have stuck to the diet and am steadily losing weight. I feel a lot better, too, mainly because I am finally doing something constructive about the state of my body – something that I feel is more sustainable and long-term than anything I tried before.

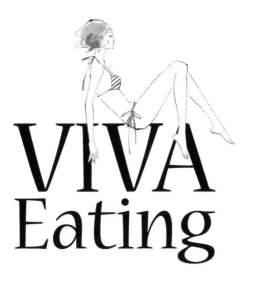

VIVA
Eating

You are about to discover:

How to eat the Viva Mayr way

How to prepare yourself mentally for the
Viva Mayr Diet

The good foods with which you can now
fill your kitchen

How to put the famous Viva Mayr spelt
bread to good use

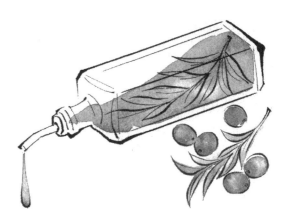

Today's Menu

Breakfast
Green tea, spelt bread, and fresh vegetable sticks with herbal spread (see page 233)

Lunch
Leafy salad with walnuts, apples and linseed dressing, and potato and vegetable gratin with spinach sauce (see page 234)

Dinner
Poached trout with vegetables and lemongrass (see page 235)

By the time you've finished this chapter and inwardly 'digested' all of the information it contains, you will have the tools you need to change your eating habits for life. This is not a complicated process. Even I managed it and I have spent most of my life just eating whatever happens to come my way. I am not the kind of person who really thinks about what I am putting into my body. Until now, that is. Meeting Dr Stossier has made me realise that leaving my body's nutrition to fate or convenience – or whatever you like to call it – is close to criminal. How can I expect my body and face to stay healthy and young if I don't even feed it properly?

Although the Viva Mayr Diet is very much focused on *how* we eat (which we will deal with in the subsequent chapters), before you can think about that, you need to decide *what* to eat.

This is where good digestion begins and, as good digestion equals slimness, youthful looks and a healthy lifestyle, it's extremely important. We are all masters of what we put in our mouths. In other words, we all have choices. No one is force-feeding us. As Dr Stossier puts it; 'If you want to go down the junk food route, then that's your decision. If you decide to opt for a healthier life that's your decision, too.' And we both know which one he would prefer us to choose.

Years ago, one nutritionist said to me that 'healthy eating begins in the supermarket'. Pretty basic, but something we tend to ignore as we pop a few 'treats' into the trolley. We all have our weak points. I have a total thing for shortbread biscuits, which I obviously don't tell Dr Stossier about, for fear of being sacked before I even begin to work on his book. But as I prepare to go for a stay at his famous Viva Mayr Clinic to research this book, I wonder if I will be searched on my way in and what may be the consequences of hiding one packet of M&S Organic shortbread fingers in my luggage. They are organic, after all.

Food provides our bodies with nutrition. Different foods provide the body with the substances it needs to live; in other words, they convey life. In order for them to give us life and health, they need to contain nutrients as well as their life force and vitality. These nutrients are defined by the quality of the food we choose to eat. So what should we be eating? Probably not shortbread biscuits. Even organic ones.

Our nutrition is divided into three groups: proteins, carbohydrates and fats. I have heard this countless times, but have no idea what it means or what I am supposed to do with this knowledge. I have also been told that we should be eating around 50–55 per cent carbohydrates, 15 per cent protein, and 30 per cent fat. Also important is fibre. So what does this all mean?

Counting carbs

'We have been told to eat more carbohydrates so that we produce energy,' says Dr Stossier. 'But really these guidelines are misguided. If we eat a lot of carbohydrates, the pancreas needs to produce a great deal of insulin to bring them into our cells. Insulin is required to metabolise carbs, and to use the energy with which they can provide us. So basically, when you eat a lot of carbs, your body converts them into sugars. In order to control your blood-sugar level, your body produces the hormone insulin. But if there is insulin in our bodies, it tell us, 'there is energy – we have enough, so use it'. So our body turns any excess energy from the carbs into fat, which is effectively a 'store' of energy for later use. It's not a great situation. As long as insulin levels remain high in the body, we will also store the other components of food, such as protein or fat. This has a massive influence on our weight, and affects the way that we should exercise as well (see page 79).

Dr Stossier suggests that we should eat about the same amount of protein but increase our intake of the right kinds of fats (making sure we make the right choices between saturated and unsaturated fatty acids; more on that later) and cut down the carbs, as well as the amount we eat overall. 'Some people eat up to 3,700 calories or more a day,' says Dr Stossier. 'This would be ideal for an active sportsman training for a competition, but it is way too much for most normally active people. There is no mystery to losing weight; cut down on carbohydrates and increase your intake of unsaturated fatty acids.'

If you think about the fact that a Krispy Kreme Caramel Kreme Crunch doughnut, or its cousin the Apple Fritter, each contains almost 400 calories a pop, you'll see how easy it is for the calories to add up. After all, who can stop at one when they sell them in handy boxes of a dozen?

The fact is that we do all eat way too much. I know I do. There is no reason at all to eat a huge breakfast and three-course lunch, and then repeat the ritual in the evening. We will go into eating in a later chapter, but it's worth noting now that since I met Dr Stossier, I sometimes skip dinner altogether and make do with a snack like some oatcakes and cream cheese. And you know what? I don't die of starvation during the night …

Not surprisingly, Dr Stossier recommends we avoid the likes of the Caramel Kreme Crunch and try to stick to organic food (see pages 50–51). I suddenly feel quite smug about my organic shortbread biscuits.

Dr Stossier doesn't like to break our diet down into percentages. He believes that if we focus on fresh fruit and vegetables (some of them raw, and at the right time), and good-quality proteins and fats, we really won't be hungry enough to fill ourselves with carbohydrates – and, in particular, the unhealthy types, such as those made with white flour and lots of sugar. When you are eating the Viva Mayr way, it's important simply to cut down on carbs by taking much smaller portions, and choosing wholegrain varieties which fill you up.

Fats

Fats are also important to overall health, and are an essential part of the Viva Mayr Diet. But fats are not all created equal. As you would on any healthy diet, it's important to avoid the unhealthy saturated types – in particular hydrogenated fats or trans fats, which are now known to cause a wide range of health problems, including heart disease and obesity. Whole, fresh milk, cream and butter are fine, because they are natural products that contain healthy fats. But avoid very fatty cuts of meat (particularly those that are processed), as well as anything that has the word 'hydrogenated' on the label – many margarines included! The very best fats you can eat are found in cold-pressed oils, and it is these fats that can not only help to keep you healthy, but *improve* your overall health and well-being immeasurably. Paradoxically, they can help you to *lose* weight – something that we might not normally attribute to oils!

Essential oils

An essential part of a healthy diet is oil. And this is the one thing you shouldn't compromise on. This must always be cold-pressed, preferably virgin, most definitely organic, and of the best quality you can find. And don't worry about oil being fattening. Unsaturated fatty acids in oils taken in their pure form are not going to make you fat.

Oils, such as linseed and olive, are an essential element of the Viva Mayr Diet, and should be eaten on a daily basis. This may seem strange, as most of us were reared on the idea that fats are unhealthy and, well, fattening, but bear with me. These oils are rich in fatty acids which are crucial to good health in many ways, and they are known as 'omega oils'. At present we have identified three of these oils, which are omega 3, omega 6 and omega 9; each is important, but it is the balance between them that is most crucial. For example, inflammatory diseases, such as arthritis, inflammation of the digestive system, and even MS, are the result of an imbalance between omega 3 and omega 6. Omega 3 oils are found in linseed oil, hemp oil, and oily fish (fish from cold, deep seas such as herring, tuna, salmon and cod) so try to add as much of those as you can to your diet. Several studies relate heart disease to a lack of omega 3. Eskimos have one of the lowest rates of heart disease due to the high levels of omega 3 fatty acids they consume. In order to benefit we need to eat them regularly.

Good sources of omega 6 oils include poultry, wholegrains, eggs, nuts, most vegetables oils, hemp and linseed oils, and even the acai berry. We tend to get enough of these in a healthy diet, which is why it's important to bump up our intake of the omega 3s, to ensure that the balance is right. And that's one reason why you'll find oils, such as linseed (flax) and hemp are widely used in the Viva Mayr Diet; their omega-3 content is crucial to overall health and wellbeing.

Omega 9 is not strictly an essential oil because our bodies can manufacture a small amount, provided we have adequate omega 3 and 6 in our diet. However, omega 9 can lower cholesterol levels, reduce the risk of cardiovascular disease, protect against certain types of cancer, improve blood-sugar balance, and encourage healthy immunity, so if you aren't getting enough of the other omegas, do ensure you get some omega 9s in your diet as well. Good sources are olive oil, olives, avocados, almonds, sesame seeds (and oil) and most nuts.

These omega oils, otherwise known as unsaturated fatty acids, are also essential for keeping you slim. The more you increase your intake of them, the less saturated fatty acids you will eat, and the less weight you will pile on around your stomach and hips. The reason for this is that the body tends to store unhealthy fats around the waist, giving us the unhealthy 'apple' shape. Omega oils (omega 3, in particular) have been found to encourage fat-burning in our bodies. In a nutshell, if you substitute omega oils for unhealthy saturated fats (such as trans fats), you will not only avoid putting on weight around your middle and hips, but you'll encourage your body to burn off what's there.

Increasing fatty acids will also boost your brain power. The brain is comprised of concentrated fatty acids. In particular, there are a lot of omega 3 fatty acids in the brain; there, they create molecules which act as transmitters. The more transmitters or pathways you have firing, the more active your thinking process becomes. This is why fish is famously good for the brain. Our ability to concentrate, our energy levels, and a well-functioning nervous system are all related to the quantity of healthy oils in our diet.

'We grew up with a teaspoon of cod liver oil,' says Dr Stossier. 'Now we are seriously lacking the omega 3 oils that it once provided every day.' Personally I didn't grow up with a teaspoon of cod liver oil, thankfully, but maybe I would be healthier if I had?

What to buy?

Oils are the first things to put on your shopping list when you begin the Viva Mayr Diet. You need three types of oils for the three types of omegas. Unsaturated vegetable oil, such as olive oil, will provide you with omega 9, hemp or linseed oil is a great source of omega 3 oils; and you can choose sunflower or other nut and seed oils for their omega 6 content. Take two tablespoons of one of these oils every day, making sure that you manage some linseed or hemp at least three times a week. If you don't eat fish, it's a good idea to take a good-quality fish oil supplement as well.

This is not as difficult as it sounds. Use the oils much as you do salt and pepper, and sprinkle it over whatever it is you are eating. You can swallow the two tablespoons in the morning, or mix them with some soup or even porridge. Some of them have a distinct taste, but they aren't unpleasant. There is a recipe on page 279 for Herb spread, which is delicious blended with oil. Eaten with some bread, it is perfect for breakfast, lunch or as a snack. The only rule to follow with all of these oils is to *avoid heating them*. At high temperatures, these oils become toxic. You can, however, pour them over hot food, as they would have to be heated to 60° degrees Celsius to become unhealthy trans fats. If you do wish to cook with oils such as olive, sunflower or nut oils, choose the warm-pressed varieties (see page 31).

Cold-pressed oils need to be stored away from light, air and heat because they are extremely fragile. They should be stored in dark glass bottles, ideally in a cool place, such as a refrigerator. Olive oil will solidify when it becomes very cool; however, it will soon return to liquid form at room temperature. Some olive oils are also sold in cans to protect them from light. Pay attention to the expiry date or, even better, the pressing date if listed, to know the oil's age. Once opened, cold-pressed oils should be used quickly, as they will become rancid and lose their nutritional value. Once oils have become rancid, they should no longer be used. They don't taste good, and they do more harm than good to our health.

You should also stock up on nuts and seeds, because they contain omega fatty acids in their natural form and are also full of a concentrated form of antioxidants (see pages 207–8). Try sprinkling sunflower seeds, sesame seeds and pumpkin seeds on your meals – anything from baked salmon, porridge and salad to sandwiches, puddings and even fruit tastes delicious with that little extra crunch. If you are prone to snacking, carry some nuts or seeds around with you instead of a KitKat (although Dr Stossier says that if you follow the Viva Mayr programme you won't feel the need to snack any more).

Try to get into the habit of thinking about everything you put into your mouth. Is it good for you? If not, give it a miss. If you can't hit 100 per cent, do as a friend of mine suggests, and aim for 90.

Look after your proteins

Proteins are an important part of a healthy diet, but you should avoid eating too many. In fact, Dr Stossier suggests that we should eat fish and other animal proteins, such as cheese and meat, a maximum of every second day. Better sources are vegetable proteins, such as pulses, seeds and nuts, which provide us with the amino acids we need in a more easily digested form.

'People focus too much on proteins because they think they need them to give them energy,' says Dr Stossier. 'Eating too many proteins causes our bodies to store them, which means they are not properly digested in the intestine, leading to putrification.'

Putri-*what*? It sounds disgusting. Dr Stossier explains that putrification, or 'toxin overload' as I will call it, is the result of protein being metabolised more by intestinal bacterial overgrowth than by our own digestive enzymes. This is part of a maldigestive process (we'll go into this in more detail later; see pages 127–8) that leads to a buildup of toxins in our bodies. These substances have to be eliminated by our metabolic organs (such as the liver and kidneys), or else they will be stored in connecting tissues between your bloodstream and cells. If these get blocked up, then we can't supply blood to the cells. In turn, the cells produce waste products and we can't dispose of them, so the waste products are stored. This leads to an overload of toxins, causing heart attack, strokes, rheumatic diseases, diabetes and all sorts of dreadful things. So not only do we have more toxins in our bodies, but our detoxification organs are put under enormous pressure, which compromises their ability to do their jobs effectively. If this all seems a trifle unclear (sorry to mention trifle) then fear not, it will all be explained a little later in the book. Better still, putrification can be avoided, faster than you can learn how to spell it.

To reduce the risk of a toxin overload while eating proteins, and for better digestion, white meat is best, such as turkey, veal and chicken. Lamb follows that, then red meat and last of all pork. Game is somewhere between white and red meat. All fish is fine; eel is slightly fatty, but how often do you come across that? Also bear in mind that cream cheese is more easily digestible than hard cheese (see pages 279–80 for delicious cream-cheese spreads). Some people also find goat's and sheep's cheeses easier to digest. Why? Because all milks contain a sugar called lactose. Our bodies have an enzyme known as 'lactase', which is used to digest lactose. As we get older, our bodies produce decreasing quantities of this enzyme, which means that we may find it harder and harder to digest milk and milk products. Goat's and sheep's milk contains less lactose, so can often be more easily tolerated. And, again, other good sources of protein include pulses (lentils, dried beans and peas, for example), and nuts and seeds. In fact, many other foods, including potatoes, contain some protein, as well as whole grains. So you will be getting more than you think you are, even before you take a bite of that steak.

Don't forget your fibre

Fibre is an essential part of your diet, as it acts like a broom in the digestive system, clearing out the debris and moving the food along. Better digestion can prevent putrificaction in the gut, and it can also ensure that toxins don't hang around for ages, where they can be absorbed into the bloodstream through the walls of the intestines. What's more, fibre ensures that digestion occurs at the right speed, giving the body time to absorb the nutrients from our food. Where do you find fibre? In whole, fresh foods, such as vegetables, fruit and whole grains. Nuts and seeds will provide you with some fibre as well. You'll be getting plenty on the Viva Mayr Diet.

Many of us do not get enough fibre in our diets because we choose refined foods over the wholegrain alternatives. White bread and pasta, for example, will contain very little fibre, whereas wholegrain bread has lots. White bread is what Dr Stossier calls 'empty food', devoid or low in nutrients and not much use to our bodies.

'It is insane that people will eat white bread and then take a fibre supplement,' he says, getting almost angry. I am really beginning to see why he is nicknamed the 'friendly werewolf'. He definitely has a wolf-like quality. I am thankful it's not a full moon as he continues his tirade. 'Why not just eat some brown bread and get the job done?'

Furthermore, make sure you choose wholemeal cereals, wholemeal noodles and pasta, muesli, oats and so forth, whenever possible.

Eating your greens… and reds, yellows, purples…

Other foods that you should make a beeline for when shopping are brightly coloured fruits and vegetables. The bright colour signifies a large number of antioxidants, which they will pass on to us (see page 50), and fresh vegetables and fruit are also rich in a variety of other vitamins and minerals, as well as being a very good source of fibre. We'll talk about antioxidants a little later (see pages 207–8); however, for now, you may want to know that they are, for one thing, the nutrients that can help slow down the degenerative effects of ageing. I can't think of anyone who wouldn't want some of those! Remember that fruit and vegetables will contain fewer antioxidants if they are not grown in a natural environment. You'll be getting plenty of fresh and raw vegetables and fruit on the Viva Mayr Diet. What's more important here, however, is when you eat them.

Going organic

The reason for choosing organic food and drink is that humans take energy from food, energy that is produced by the sun. This energy was first measured by a man called Professor Fritz Popp (I promise you, that is his real name) and it is called a 'biophoton', from the Greek word meaning life and light. A tomato that has been exposed to plenty of sunshine has a lot more of the kind of energy we need than one that was forced in a greenhouse in winter. This is because a tomato that has been grown naturally will be full of antioxidants, which it has had to produce in order to protect it from the negative effects of the sun. These are the very same antioxidants that we can use to protect our bodies. In fact, there is some recent research that suggests that skin creams that contain antioxidants enhance the protection they give to our skin.

'Take an orange, for example,' says Dr Stossier. 'It gets its nutrients from the soil; it grows and produces its fruit under the influence of sunlight and a natural environment. The life force, or 'energy' of a plant is contained within it, and when we eat that plant, we also take in its energy. This is measurable, and is known as a 'bioprotein'. So, a bioprotein is, in fact, a measurement of a food's vitality, or energy. And studies have found that organic food contains many more of these bioproteins than non-organic food. Organic food does give us much more vitality than other foods, so wherever possible you should buy organic.

It makes sense to eat food that is as natural as possible. Not only is it healthier, but it also mirrors our own natural state. Unfortunately, some production processes either prevent the food's energy from being created (for example, if it has no access to natural sunlight) or destroy it (for example, by irradiating food to preserve it or cooking food in a microwave oven).'

There are a multitude of other reasons to eat organic, including supporting sustainable farming, ensuring we aren't consuming unhealthy pesticides, herbicides, growth hormones, and other chemicals in our food, and avoiding GMOs (genetically modified organisms), which may contain little or no vitality at all.

Having said that, eating organic is not the most important aspect of the Viva Mayr philosophy, and if you don't have access to organic food there are many things you can do to compensate. 'Apart from the really obvious things like junk food and sweets with no nutritional value, there is nothing you have to avoid as long as you chew it properly,' says Dr Stossier. 'Food is not good or bad, food is food; it is neutral. It is always a question of what we can get out of the food, so we have to look at our eating habits. The quality of the food is not the most important thing, but if we can reduce the intake of industrially prepared foods then it's a good thing.'

So I guess shortbread biscuits are out? Unless they are homemade? 'They lack nutritional value,' says Dr Stossier, smiling. All very well, but they have many other things going for them.

The Viva Mayr Diet is not about depriving yourself, but about eating the right thing at the right time and optimising your digestive capacity, which in turns leads to a healthier, slimmer, less-prone-to-ageing you. In fact, what you eat is not nearly as important as when you eat it. But do try to stick to the menu plans outlined on each day of the programme, or investigate some of the alternative recipes at the back of the book (see page 278–81). Enjoy experimenting with things you may never have tried before. A shift in your eating habits is the ultimate goal, and you'll soon find you are feeling better than you ever have before.

In summary ...

- Eat less – we all eat much more than we need to.

- Focus on eating more fats (choosing cold-pressed oils), and fewer carbohydrates, which will lead to healthier digestion, and overall good health.

- Eat animal proteins – meat and fish – only every second day.

- Remember that good eating begins in the supermarket – don't think for even one second that if you buy a packet of jaffa cakes you won't eat them.

- Avoid 'empty' foods – there is no point in eating white bread and then taking a fibre supplement.

- Only fry food in warm-pressed oils. Virgin or cold-pressed oils become toxic when heated at high temperatures.

- Go organic whenever you can, but don't get overly stressed about it.

- Remember it only takes a few days to break bad habits forever.

Case Study

Rachel, 28, Stevenage

I used to be a junk-food junkie. I couldn't walk past a McDonald's without salivating. I would start the day with breakfast on the run – either a doughnut or almond croissant or something similarly sweet. I always needed a sugar rush. And, of course, I would drink coffee to help wake me up, too. Lunch would normally be McDonald's or Pizza Hut. By the end of the day I felt faintly sick, but I sort of got used to it, and then I would go out and have lots of wine after work. This way of eating and drinking started when I was 18 and a student. I guess at that age your body can almost handle it, but the older I got the more unhealthy I started to feel. I also, understandably, put on weight. I couldn't face doing any exercise because I felt so dreadful.

New Year's last year was a turning point. I tried on every dress in my wardrobe but had the most awful VPL with every one. Then I realised it wasn't the VPL that was the problem – it was my bum that was the problem. I went out and got drunk, but made one big resolution: to change my eating habits and do some exercise. A friend of mine had been to the Viva Mayr Clinic and told me about the diet, about eating a big breakfast, chewing well, eating organic and avoiding all the things I had been eating.

The first week was the worst. I swear I was in withdrawal. I longed for some stodge, but I had promised myself to totally avoid anything like that. I started with muesli and thought I was going to throw up. I had to chew it about 40 times to be able to swallow it! I ate fruit in the morning, too, which tasted bitter to me, used as I was to sugar-coated doughnuts. For lunch I would buy a salad or something. By mid-afternoon on the second day I had headaches and felt faint, as well as hungry! I kept motivating myself by thinking about how I would soon fit into my clothes and start to feel better. In fact, I started to look better almost straight away. My skin became clearer almost overnight and my eyes sparkled.

On the third day I woke up full of energy and almost (not quite!) looking forward to my muesli. I didn't feel depressed at the thought of not eating a doughnut on my way to the office. I actually enjoyed eating rocket salad and parmesan with a piece of grilled chicken when I went out for lunch. Actually, I think day three was a turning point. I really was amazed at how quickly it had all happened — how ten years of bad eating had been changed almost overnight. OK, so I wasn't totally off junk food — I still had enormous cravings for it — but the results I had seen already made me go on and made me strong. It's true that when I went to the supermarket I practically had to shut my eyes when going past the Pringles, but I made it and was very proud of myself.

Almost like a drug addict, I told myself I had to have a whole month off junk food to really clean out my system. At the end of that month I would allow myself a treat. During those first few days that treat was the only light in a dark tunnel. But, oddly enough, at the end of my month I had totally and utterly lost the craving for junk food. I even went to McDonald's the day after my month was up and the smell, which used to get my gastric juices going, made me feel sick!

I am not a saint and I am still not quite as healthy as I would like to be, but that excess weight fell off. This all happened four months ago and I am still going strong. I am happier, healthier, thinner and more determined than ever to keep eating the Viva Mayr way.

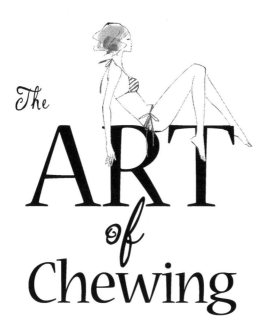

The ART of Chewing

You are about to discover:

Why you need to eat slowly and chew your food properly

How to chew your food properly

Why chewing is the single most important thing you can do for your digestion and general health

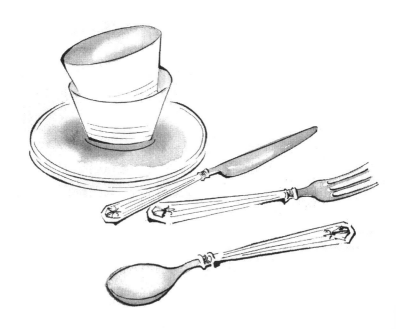

Today's Menu

Breakfast
Rosemary tea, spelt bread, vegetable spread and half an avocado (see page 280)

Lunch
Courgette soup, and grilled chicken on hash-browned potatoes and vegetables with fresh herb oil (see pages 236–7)

Dinner
Buckwheat blinis with vegetable cubes (see page 238)

The focus of today's chapter is chewing; one of the pillars of the Viva Mayr Diet, and possibly its most crucial element. If you take one thing away with you from this book it should be the ability to chew your food properly.

Chewing properly is the key to the Viva Mayr way, and also the key to losing weight quickly, and encouraging overall health and well-being. When you chew more, you eat less because your brain sends signals telling you that you've had enough. This means you get thinner faster. It also means you eat less because the nutrients from the food are absorbed more effectively, and your body craves less food to live on. What's more, chewing efficiently and for the right length of time encourages your body to absorb the nutrients in your food, which means you'll be getting far more from the food you eat, which enhances your health on all levels.

OK. This is it. This is where the Viva Mayr Diet begins in earnest. This is the morning routine you will follow for today, for the rest of the diet and, hopefully, the rest of your life. Are you ready? You're going to feel great at the end of today – you're going to experience a real sense of achievement, a feeling that you are finally doing something positive about your weight and your health.

You will have started your day with a cup of water – hot or at room temperature. Drink this half an hour before breakfast (which will give you the chance to read the rest of the chapter or go for a shower). In the next chapter we'll introduce you to some stretching exercises, but for now just gently try to touch your toes, then come up, vertebrae by vertebrae. Stretch your arms high up in the air, then stretch back down again.

Learning to chew

Now that you are feeling limber and refreshed, it's time to get to grips with the art of chewing. Dr Stossier says that if you concentrate it should take you about three weeks to learn to chew properly. It might take even less. Let's start straight away with breakfast. You may want to get up slightly earlier so that you can take longer over this crucial meal.

Begin with some bread that you prepared yesterday. If you haven't had a chance to make the famous Viva Mayr spelt bread, then purchase some spelt or rye bread from your local health-food shop, which is rich in fibre and whole grains. These are good for your digestion, and encourage you to chew because they are denser than most commercially prepared breads. If all else fails, get a good-quality wholegrain bread from your supermarket.

Take a small piece of bread and put it in your mouth, and then slowly start chewing it. Focus on keeping it there as long as possible. If you're anything like me it will disintegrate within about seven chews. Persevere, take another piece and start again. You'll find that you become more adept at keeping the bread in your mouth, and eventually you will taste a sweetness that is the result of the carbohydrates turning to sugar. Move the bread around your mouth.

Now try the chewing exercise over a whole meal. Start with your breakfast, and continue to focus on your chewing for every meal throughout the day. They are all good chewing material!

 You will notice that the Viva Mayr Diet is not an exclusion diet. It is not about cutting things out, like dairy products and wheat; rather, it is about learning how to eat them so they are easy to digest and therefore don't cause you any problems.

Savour every mouthful

Take a small piece of your breakfast spelt (or other) bread and put it in your mouth. Really savour it. Remember that it needs to be totally disintegrated before you swallow it. Try to think about what it is you are eating, and the nutrients you are putting into your body. During breakfast you can take a little bit of herbal or green tea by the spoonful, but no water (the reasons for this will be explained a little later).

Eat some herbal spread with your bread, adding it to your mouth when you have chewed the bread, to mix it with the saliva you have produced. Swallow when your food is liquid.

Next start on the scrambled eggs. If you wish, you can toast your spelt bread and serve the eggs on top. Focus on achieving a real taste sensation, which only comes after extensive chewing. Keep moving the toast (or bread) and eggs around your mouth to avoid swallowing before you've reached at least 30 chews. Eventually you will taste a total mix of all of the elements, but it's important to *really* taste the bread and the eggs. It is an intoxicating feeling and will motivate you to keep going. Later on in the book, when you move on to eating muesli for breakfast, you should aim to experience a similar sensation – savouring and really tasting the sweetness of the berries, the crunchiness of the grains and nuts, and the rich taste of whatever milk you choose.

Aim for 40 chews

Dr Stossier says he chews every mouthful between 30 and 40 times, at every meal. So it could be helpful to count at the beginning of your chewing training, to get you into the rhythm of it. At first you will only manage around 15, but this soon improves. Dr Stossier insists that chewing is one of the most crucial things you can do, because if you don't get the hang of this, nothing else will work. As he puts it, 'Forgetting to chew in your mouth and expecting your stomach to chew your food instead is not an option.'

I ask him if his children follow his chewing example.

'They are more or less trained,' he says smiling. And it *is* all about training. You can do it, just as you can train yourself to do 20 press-ups every morning.

Improving your chewing technique

Really think about chewing for the rest of the day, at lunch and at dinner. Aim to chew each mouthful between 30 and 40 times, if you possibly can. At the beginning you'll need to keep count. It will seem like an eternity because, if you're anything like me, you are probably used to swallowing your food practically whole. After just a day, though, you will start to see a change. When I first tried chewing for so long it seemed impossible, but after just two days I found I was almost chewing more without thinking and without having to concentrate so hard. In fact, after a few days I looked back with shame and slight disgust on all my years of throwing food in and swallowing before I'd even thought about it.

Before swallowing, try to sense how the food feels in your mouth. Are there still big chunks of food, and above all, has the food's taste changed? You must never swallow anything that has a recognisable shape. Sorry if this sounds gross, but it's true. If you can still identify a food, then your stomach will have to work far too hard to break it down into a digestible form. Step by step, try to chew long enough to turn the food in your mouth into a liquid before swallowing. This is a challenge, but remember it is the best thing you can do for your health and your waistline. In the early stages it will be difficult to do this in company, unless you're willing to talk with your mouth full almost constantly.

Dr Stossier sees eating as almost akin to meditation. 'When was the last time you really thought about what you are eating?' he asks. 'The last time you totally focused on the taste, the shape, the colour, the consistency of every mouthful? Try to give the food, and the preparer, the respect they deserve and think about it.'

If you can't face staring into thin air, read a book, but avoid anything depressing or stressful. As you will see from Day

Eleven, it is important to eat in a stress-free environment. This requires motivation and patience. Don't say 'I can't do it' and give up. It really is worth it, and you really can do it. It's simply a matter of making the choice to do so. Just as a woman can never be too thin or a man too rich, you can never chew too much. This is something I learned while watching clients at Dr Stossier's Viva Mayr Clinic.

Although you can very easily learn to chew properly at home, I was lucky enough to be able to head off to Austria to crack the chewing thing.

Chew your way to a thinner you

It's amazing that a simple thing like chewing your food properly can have such a dramatic effect. Although Dr Mayr was the first medical man to record its importance, the concept of purposeful chewing really started with a man called Horace Fletcher – or 'The Great Masticator', as he became known – who was born in 1849. His catchphrase was, 'Nature will castigate those who don't masticate', and he argued that every mouthful should be chewed at least 32 times. Not only would this increase a person's strength, he believed, but it would also reduce the amount they ate. It might sound wacky, but as a result of promoting his theories on lecture tours, Horace became a millionaire.

When Dr Stossier massaged my inflamed intestines in order to ease the congestion going on in there, he explained the physiological reasons why chewing food well is so important. First of all, taking time to chew means that we eat less. According to Dr Stossier, we all eat far too much anyway.

'Chewing a lot sends signals to the brain telling it that you have had enough,' he says. 'So the first thing chewing more will do is make you healthier, as well as encouraging you to lose weight by reducing your food intake.'

This stands to reason, as we are creatures of habit. Somewhere deep in our subconscious there must be something telling the brain when we've had enough, and this must in part be regulated by how many times we have chewed.

The second reason is that our digestive system begins at our lips. With our lips we feel the food, we assess the texture, and we send signals to our brain to let it know what it can expect. While you are recognising taste, the brain is also hard at work. When we chew our food properly the brain recognises the ingredients it contains, which provides our digestive system (more specifically the pancreas and the liver) with important information for preparing the digestive juices needed to digest whatever is on its way down. Protein requires different digestive juices than carbohydrates or fats. Chewing is important because it gives advance notice to our digestive system to start the appropriate programmes for subsequent chemical digestion. This, in turn, eases the pressure on the digestive system.

Our mouths are essential to healthy nutrition because this is where we use our teeth to chop and grind foods mechanically, and to break them into small pieces. Insufficient chewing at this stage will mean the whole digestive system has to work so much harder to metabolise the food. And it could also mean we are missing out on the goodness of the food we eat.

Yet another reason why chewing well is so important is because it helps us to produce more saliva. Saliva is not something I think about a lot. In fact, I prefer not to think about it. And I haven't talked about it since my school days when we swapped stories about snogging boys. Even then, less was always more. Now more is very definitely acceptable. Saliva is crucial to our digestive system for two main reasons. For one thing, it mixes with the food in our mouths to begin that all-important digestive process. Saliva contains enzymes needed to process carbohydrates, and starts the digestion of starches and sugars in the mouth. If you chew bread or pasta really well, for example, you will find that they begin to taste slightly sweet as the carbohydrates turn to sugar. Until you get that sweet taste, you haven't chewed enough.

The digestive process requires the finely tuned cooperation of all participating organs. One function depends upon the function of another. It is obvious that bits that are done incorrectly in one phase cannot be made up later in the process. Chewing happens in the mouth and if it is not done well, this lack of mechanical processing cannot be compensated for later. This creates problems for the subsequent digestive processes. It's time to adapt your personal eating habits to nature's requirements and not the other way around. Well chewed is half-digested, as the friendly werewolf puts it.

'If you buy an organic salad and you wolf it down quickly, you will not reap the benefits from it,' said Dr Stossier, as he kneaded my large intestine during the initial consultation. (And by the way, have you noticed how fond he is of the word wolf? Should I be worried?)

'In fact,' he said, 'You may gain more benefit from a Big Mac with a single salad leaf in it if it is chewed properly.' This was amazing news to me.

'So just by chewing something properly we increase its nutritional value several times?' I asked.

He nodded. 'Yes, there is no point in spending money on organic food and then not chewing it properly. You may as well be eating something processed.'

Chew for your brain

There is another important point to make about chewing. We originally thought that the number of brain cells cannot be increased, and that it is the *number* of cells that count when it comes to brain functioning. This has been found to be totally wrong. We now know that brain cells can build connections to other cells, and send information through these connections. And it is possible to continue to build these connections throughout our lives. We are constantly creating neural pathways that keep the brain active. The more we use them, the better the connection; and, similarly, if we fail to use them, they close down. Most importantly, perhaps, we should aim to create *new* connections whenever possible, by doing things slightly differently, or choosing to do things we have never done before. For example, even if you hate modern music, you could make an effort to listen to it in order to create new connections and pathways. Creating new routes in our brain is an important way of staving off degenerative diseases such as Alzheimer's.

The second brain

'We have a second brain in the stomach,' said Dr Stossier. 'There are exactly the same number of nerve cells there as there are in the brain.' And the intestine also has the same transmitter functions as the brain. Our brains work when we use our stomachs, and what is true for the brain is also true for the stomach. The only time we have control over it, the only time we can use it to create connections, is when food is in our mouth. So we need to take greater advantage of our mouths than we do now. For example, the length of time we chew will affect the function of our livers and our pancreas, and in that way a new pathway is created. Practising chewing is, in fact, training for the digestion that is going on in other parts of our intestines.

Breaking bad habits

Unlearning bad chewing habits takes about three to four weeks, according to Dr Stossier. This is nothing if you compare it to how long you've been gulping down your food too quickly. My husband, for example, used to be annoy me by eating too quickly – even before I met Dr Stossier. I remember once, relatively early in our relationship, asking him why he always wolfed his food.

'It's the result of being brought up with two older brothers,' he told me. 'If I didn't eat everything immediately they would.'

I tried to point out that his brothers were now unlikely to be lurking around every corner waiting for him to miss a roast potato. But it was no good, this was a habit he had grown up with, and it would take more than that to erase it. Obviously once he's read this book, he'll be a changed man!

Less is more

When I left my consultation with Dr Stossier, I was hungrier than ever, and headed to the dining room full of anticipation. My taxi friend Brenda was already there, eating what looked like a piece of stale bread. She seemed very cheerful, so I assumed it couldn't be. I was shown to a table for two, where a girl called Annie would be joining me.

I was shown a menu with all sorts of things called 'spreads', and I opted for one called Salmon and Avocado. I imagined a spread of beautifully sliced avocado and smoked salmon with a slice of lemon on the side and maybe some olive oil. Then I was handed a piece of bread, and it did feel slightly stale. I took a bite. It was stale. But I was now so hungry I couldn't stop eating it.

Annie joined me. She was young, pretty and thin. Why was she here? Was she a spy for Dr Stossier, sent in to make sure we didn't sneak anything untoward onto our plates, like that shortbread biscuit that was lurking in my towelling robe pocket?

'I have been feeling dreadful for months,' she told me. 'Turns out I have candida. I am on a potato diet.'

'Just potato?'

'Pretty much, for the first few days, that is. How about you?'

'I'm allowed most things at the moment, I think, I've just ordered some salmon and avocado,' I told her.

Annie looked amazed. A bowl of boiled potatoes arrived for her with a sprig of dill on top.

'You should slow down with that bread, by the way,' she said, picking up her fork. 'The idea is to chew every mouthful about 40 times.'

Of course! I have just had a lecture about this. So this was it; the first challenge, the first step to a new, slim, healthy, gorgeous me. I bit off a piece of bread and chewed it. After seven chews it was gone – already on its way down to join the traffic jam in my small intestine. Or was it the large one? I was about 33 chews light. What the hell was going on?

'You get used to it,' said Annie, who had still not started eating her very tempting potatoes. 'You have to move it around your mouth. It takes practice.'

'What if I just take a bigger bite?' I suggested.

'No,' said Annie, slowly chewing a piece of potato. 'You're meant to take small bites.'

I tried again. This time it was better. I managed about 16

chews before the piece of stale bread totally disintegrated. I was looking forward to my salmon, that's for sure. I had almost finished my stale bread (which was actually called spelt bread and has a rather nice spicy aftertaste) and was still hungry. The waitress arrived with what looked like an egg-cup full of cream cheese, which she put down in front of me.

'No, no,' I protested. 'I ordered a spread of salmon and avocado and all sorts of things. This must be for Annie.'

The waitress looked at me in a stern manner. 'Annie is only eating potatoes. This is the spread.'

OK, I got it. So the spread was actually a cheese spread with salmon and avocado in it. Great. What was for dinner? I considered nicking one of Annie's potatoes, but that would be mean. And as I was going to be sitting with her for the next six days it might not be such a smart move.

Lucky I have my sneaky shortbread biscuits for pudding.

I took a mouthful of the spread. It was totally delicious – soft, creamy, tasty. Shame I didn't have any bread left to go with it. Annie was still munching her way through her potatoes. I had never seen anyone chew so much, but then I guess that's what we were there for.

The (in)famous Viva Mayr spelt bread

When you eat your dinner of soup and spelt bread, make sure that you chew well and try to as do as follows:

- Take one bite of the spelt bread, and chew that bit 30 to 50 times.

- Take a small spoonful of the soup and chew it together a few times.

- Swallow.

- Repeat that process.

- Add the spread in the same way.

- Stop as soon as you feel you've had enough.

The aim of the spelt bread, Dr Stossier, explained to me later on, is to re-train your body to chew properly. And it's not just a health issue, it's a question of taste. Taste only develops in the mouth if sufficient saliva is available. Saliva forms chemical bonds with foods that our taste buds are then able to sense. Our taste buds are special areas in the mouth, primarily on the tongue, but also in the mucous membranes of our cheeks and throat. These taste buds sense a chemical reaction and forward this information via our nervous system to a central location that connects these taste sensations with our experience. This enables us to recognise if a food tastes good, which flavour components are present – sweet, sour, bitter or salty – and even if the food is rotten and should be spat out.

So if you want to enjoy your food, chew it properly. What is the point in paying double for an organic tomato and then neither reaping the nutritional benefits nor tasting it? There is also a weight loss element that should be considered. If you *really* taste your food, you are unlikely to eat so much food that is bad for you. What's more, junk food will lose it's appeal. You will crave healthy, fresh food that tastes good and keeps you slim.

Top tips for chewing properly

Breathe, take it slowly, and relax.

Put down your cutlery between each mouthful.

Try eating your meals with chopsticks, which will slow you down and ensure you take smaller mouthfuls.

If you're eating hot food, make sure your plate is heated or your food will get cold.

Just when you think you've finished chewing, bring the food to a different area of the mouth and start again.

Take a pause between each mouthful.

Make sure you take *at least* half an hour over every meal.

Look at people around you, and watch how quickly they swallow their food. It will inspire you to change.

Do some of the training with covered eyes to see if you can recognise what you're eating; what food is it and how does it taste?

Think about what you're putting in your mouth; anticipate the flavours and the texture.

Do not swallow until your food is in liquid form.

Chewing fills you up

I felt I'd made progress even after my first meal at the Viva Mayr Clinic. Strangely enough I didn't even feel hungry after my meagre dinner. I decided to save my shortbread biscuits for another day. I bumped into Dr Stossier on my way to my room, and told him how pleased I was to have started the chewing thing.

'It is one of those things that once you start thinking about it,' he said encouragingly, 'it really comes naturally. In fact, it seems crazy that you ever did it any other way. Especially when you see the list of all the benefits of chewing properly.'

After three days of chewing properly I definitely felt the benefits. I felt thinner (I was eating less), more energetic and I had no feelings of bloating, or that awful feeling of eating too much and wanting to do nothing but go to sleep as soon as I have eaten. I could see how chewing could become a habit you can't break and I was really pleased that I had adopted it before I created a seriously damaging situation in my stomach. The shortbread biscuits remained untouched – I was saving them for an emergency.

The benefits of chewing your food properly

You will increase the amount and quality of saliva you produce. This means optimal preparation for subsequent digestion, because you have more saliva and because the increased saliva production provides information to the brain about the food ingested and the required digestion processes.

You will taste everything you eat, which means that you will be naturally attracted to healthier foods because they taste better.

It is good exercise for the jaw, which means you don't end up with that very ageing jowly look.

Chewing more also means you are making optimal use of the food you eat, which leads to eating less.

Putting it into practice

Since I left the clinic I have more or less kept up with the chewing. Of course I have lapses and there are times when I simply don't have the time to chew properly, but they are now few and far between, I really make an effort to make chewing a priority.

Now I make sure that I have a proper breakfast. If it looks as though I'm running out of time I blend a juice of fresh fruit or vegetables that doesn't need chewing, and which can be sipped slowly while I drive to work. Clearly it would be better to sit down at the table, but sometimes that just isn't going to happen. If I'm really hungry I sometimes find myself wolfing food down (love using that word) but it only takes a minute for me to realise what I'm doing and stop. In fact looking at other people wolfing down food is one of the most inspirational things you can do. It's a bit like when you give up smoking and watch someone inhaling poison into their lungs as you sit there smugly thinking 'How could they do that?' Watching someone shovel food into their mouth has the same effect on me. 'Their poor digestive system,' I find myself thinking, and I'm often tempted to go up to them and explain what they're doing to themselves. But they would probably tell me, with a mouthful of food, to mind my own business.

But it was really only a few nights ago that I realised just how amazing the whole chewing thing is. We had some friends over for dinner. I made fresh pasta. I have a very special relationship with pasta. Being half-Italian, I tend to eat about twice as much as I should. I have never sat down to eat pasta and not taken second and even third and fourth helpings. Imagine my horror then the other night when my lovingly handmade Fettucine Alfredo was vanishing before my eyes. Early on in the dinner, it was clear to me by the way the guests were raving about it that they would want seconds. And as I was the hostess, it was a case of FHB (or 'Family Hold Back'). I decided there was only one thing for it: Chew. So I chewed meticulously. Dr S would have been proud of me. I might even have outchewed him. By the time the friend sitting next to me had finished her plate and was heading for seconds, I had only eaten half of mine. Incredibly, by the time my plate was empty (and the large bowl with the pasta in it was, too), I no longer wanted seconds. It was a first for me, and a milestone for the new Viva Mayr me.

In summary ....

- You need to chew each mouthful 40 times, until it is in liquid form.

- Chewing can bring you a number of benefits, which will lead to a thinner and healthier you.

Case Study

Rebecca, 47, Edinburgh

My mother always told me to chew my food properly and I always ignored her. My mind was always racing off to the next thing and the next mouthful. I would have carried on the way I always had done if I hadn't seen an article about the benefits of chewing, and how much damage we can do to ourselves if we don't chew properly. I started to look into it and came across the Viva Mayr approach to eating. It seemed to make sense to me – it was just logical and easy to understand. So I started chewing. The first few times I tried to chew 40 times I fell about laughing. I got to about seven and then the food was gone. I just couldn't see how on earth I was going to get to 40 or even 20. But I persevered and eventually got the knack of moving the food around my mouth to optimise the chewing possibilities, and making sure it really was in a liquid form before I swallowed it. If you really concentrate it is easier. It's almost a meditative process – you just have to focus on chewing and nothing else. That's why it is better to start alone if you can, or at least with someone who knows what you're up to.

I remember my first lunch out with friends as a 'chewer'. I was so much slower than them, and to begin with I was embarrassed. But when I started explaining to them what I was up to, they got really interested in it, and I was pleased to be able to tell them all about it. That's the thing, I suppose – it really does make sense. I mean, why should your stomach mash up the food? In fact, it can't, can it? That's what your teeth are for. I don't really know how or why we lost the habit of chewing, but we did, or at least I did. But now I have got back into it I am thrilled. I am thinner, more energetic and happier than ever. And I swear it is anti-ageing! My friends often comment that I am looking better than ever; maybe it's all the exercise my jowls are getting!

GETTING
Active

You are about to discover:

Why exercise is essential for your digestion, weight and general health

How to eat to make your exercising more effective

Exercise tips to keep you slim and trim

The tools you need to ensure you will never become immobile

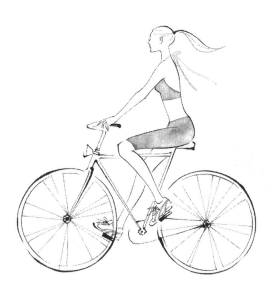

Today's Menu

Breakfast
Mallow tea, pomegranate juice, and Viva muesli with soft cheese and fresh fruit (see page 239)

Lunch
Broccoli soup, and wild salmon with spinach and carrot mash (see page 240)

Dinner
Baked potatoes with fresh herb dip (see page 241)

To digest our food well (of course it all begins with digestion for Dr Stossier!) we need to move. Voluntary muscle movements such as running and jumping help to stimulate the involuntary, internal ones that help food to move along our digestive tracts, and that's fundamental to good digestive health.

When we move, nutrients from the food we eat supply our muscles with energy. The balance between supply of energy and movement (which uses this energy) obviously affects our body weight. If we move enough in relation to how much we eat, then we stay fit and slim. If we don't, then the energy will be stored in our fat tissue.

Interestingly, though, it is not simply a question of exercising like a lunatic from dawn till dusk; in fact this can have the reverse effect to the one you're after. If you overdo it you produce a lot of lactic acid, which can block weight loss, because when your metabolism notices there is acid around it retains water to reduce the negative effects of that acid. So in a way, less can be more.

I have to admit that I quite like that muscle ache you experience after a good session in the gym – it makes me feel as though I've really worked. In fact, I used to judge the quality of a gym class by how much pain I was in the following day. But that was before I realised that the discomfort was the result of a build-up of lactic acid, which was most definitely not good for me! Granted, I still get aches sometimes if I've been to a strenuous class or started something new. When I took up Vertical Flex (as they diplomatically call it – pole-dancing to most of us), I was in agony for a whole week. I literally couldn't lift my arms. But most of the time I can't feel my muscles at all because they are used to working at the level I ask them to work.

To avoid a build-up of lactic acid (you'll learn more about this on Day Twelve) Dr S suggests making sure you don't let yourself get oxygen deficient. Take this simple test while exercising: try to say a sentence of 11 words out loud. If you don't run out of breath then you are fine.

'A little every day goes a long way,' my grandmother used to say and Dr S agrees that the key to exercise is regularity, not intensity.

He suggests exercising every second or third day for between 30 and 40 minutes. (Personally, I suggest aiming to do something every day because if you start with that aim you are more likely to make it to three or four times a week.)

'Life as we have seen is rhythmic,' says Dr Stossier. 'And regular exercise will be far more beneficial than irregular exercise, even if it is much more intensive.'

Eating to enhance the effects of exercise

We exercise to keep our heart and lungs healthy, to retain muscle tone and joint mobility, and also to help keep our weight under control (or reduce it if we're overweight). But certain types of food can undermine our exercise efforts, while other types can enhance them. Here's a quick guide to what you can eat to get the best from your exercise sessions.

First of all, you should cut down on carbs. When we eat a lot of carbs, we need to produce more of the hormone insulin to regulate the metabolism of the sugar they break down into. The more carbs we eat, the more sugar we produce and the more insulin the pancreas creates to deal with it. Excess sugars are stored as glycogen in the muscles or the liver, or converted into fat. As long as blood insulin levels stay high, we won't be able to empty these glycogen stores and burn our fat. For that, insulin levels need to be lowered – and the way to do this is to eat fewer carbs.

The general view among nutritionists is that our diet should be made up of around 55 per cent carbohydrates. Dr S believes that for a lot of people this is too high and results in a high insulin level, which makes it very difficult to lose weight.

Too much stress can also lead to situations where you are unable to shed excess weight because of its influence on our blood sugar. We'll look at stress in detail on Day Eleven but for now suffice it to say that when we are in a stressful situation, our bodies increase our blood sugar levels.

It doesn't matter what is causing your stress. Stress always blocks the metabolism, whatever the cause. Whether you have family problems or work problems, it will be more difficult to reduce your weight. Don't try to combat it by taking more exercise or reducing the amount of food you eat because that will only produce even more stress. There is a risk that your metabolism will react in the opposite way to the one you are after. Dr S tells me he often sees patients who have gained weight precisely because they started a strenuous exercise regime while they were under stress.

So you need to reduce stress in order to burn fat. In other words, don't get stressed about being overweight – nothing could be more counterproductive.

'Since so many stumbling blocks can prevent the positive effects of exercise and sports on our weight, we have to make sure we do it the right way in order to achieve our aim,' he says. 'Our approach is based on the knowledge that the muscles can use fat to metabolise energy. But that requires reducing the sugar level, because sugar is always metabolised first. This is why it is so important to reduce the amount of carbohydrates in our food.'

As we saw on Day Two, oil is not fattening per se, but it is essential in the regulation of body weight. Unsaturated fatty acids (virgin olive oil, for example) mobilise the stored fat from the tissue and activate the metabolism of fat. So they basically have a similar effect to exercise and can support your efforts to burn fat by exercising.

'Unsaturated fatty acids metabolise fat to produce more energy and, in doing so, help to reduce weight,' says Dr S.

Protein also plays an important role in exercise and weight loss – but in a completely different way. Protein is not used to produce energy primarily, but to build up our body structures, such as muscles and bones. If you haven't trained your muscles for a long time, you will have reduced muscle strength and tone. To improve your performance you will need to eat a little more protein than usual (meat, fish or cheese). But please be careful: keep it in moderation. Only Arnold Schwarzenegger needs to eat lots of protein on a daily basis.

When we start to exercise we build up muscles and burn fat at the same time so the effect might not be visible on your scales straight away. Don't be distraught (or get stressed) if the kilos don't fall off as fast as you expected, because your ratio of muscle to fat will be improving. Once you have built up the amount of muscle you need for the physical activity of your choice, the fat-burning process will begin to show on your scales. Only once this happens can you achieve your ideal weight.

And the expression 'Use it or lose it' is absolutely true. If you don't keep exercising on a regular basis, your amount of active muscles will be reduced and you may start to store fat again. That's why it's important to establish a routine – and there are several ways to do this.

Do what you enjoy

Dr S suggests that you find a type of exercise you enjoy otherwise you won't keep doing it. 'If you play sport because you have to then it will just become stressful,' he says.

We've all had that 'Oh I *must* go the gym' phrase going round in our heads – but forget that. You need to do *some* exercise but that could mean anything from pole dancing (very good for the upper body, I can highly recommend it) to walking your dog. Any form of exercise taken regularly (every second or third day) will be beneficial.

However, make sure you are working hard when you exercise. You need to be sweating lightly for the exercise to be fully effective. Dr S recommends the following:

- Aerobic exercise.
- Nordic walking (using poles for a simultaneous upper and lower body workout).
- Cycling.
- Running or jogging.
- Swimming.
- Walking, especially cross country hiking.
- Riding.
- Supervised personal training sessions.
- Weight-lifting.
- Pilates.
- Yoga.
- Ballet.
- Gymnastics.
- Team and ball sports of all kinds.

All these methods work if you do them regularly, in the right way, and keep them enjoyable.

As well as formal exercise sessions, you can introduce more strenuous movement into your day-to-day life. Take two stairs at a time, push the pram up a hill instead of taking the easy way round, really stretch and bend when you do the housework, and run with your dog instead of walking along behind.

I had an old Silver Cross pram, one of those ones with huge wheels that you probably last saw in an old film. I managed to lose my pregnancy weight through a combination of breast-feeding and pushing the Silver Cross up a particularly vicious hill near my house. The first few times I was sure I wouldn't make it, but I set myself small goals – like getting to the next tree without stopping – and gradually worked my way up until I was doing the whole hill in one. You obviously don't need a Silver Cross pram to do the same! Simply power walk wherever you are heading and clench your buttocks as you go. Push yourself to go just that little bit further or faster every day, or carry some hand weights as you walk.

There are opportunities to exercise all the time, and every little bit you do will help to create a fitter, healthier, slimmer and younger-looking you. I now make sure exercise is something I incorporate into my daily routine, just like brushing my teeth. And this is the focus on Day Four of the Viva Mayr Diet. By the end of today I hope you will be doing the same.

In summary …

- Start exercising every second or third day, to an extent where you are sweating lightly but can still speak 11 words out loud without being out of breath.

- Cut down on your carb intake, increase your consumption of the right kinds of oils, and eat a little more protein if you need to build muscle.

- A basic routine that you can do anywhere, at any time, is the secret to staying supple and slim – and looking and feeling younger.

Case Study

Margaret, 54, Brighton

If I had a penny for every time I have said, 'I must get some exercise' I would be a rich lady. I could never stick to anything at all. I would join gyms every year and go for about a month before I got fed up. I even tried alternative forms of exercise like ice-skating and riding. I couldn't stick to anything. I piled on the weight and then got even more depressed and more de-motivated. I ended up over three stone overweight, so I went to the Viva Mayr Clinic to lose it. They have a morning exercise class before breakfast. I found that once I got into the habit of stretching and moving first thing, I really liked it. I thought I would faint from hunger doing all that yoga before breakfast, but I was totally fine. I felt refreshed and energised afterwards. Now I get up every morning, have my hot water, and do some exercise at home. Some mornings I only have time for ten minutes, others I can do more, but I always do something, without fail.

I have lost two stone and have another to go, but I am well on my way. Now that I am getting thinner I am even more motivated to exercise. I have joined a Pilates class, which I go to once a week. I learned that you don't have to sweat to burn fat or tone your muscles. Some of the moves we do in Pilates are really difficult, even if we're practically lying still. I would say to anyone just start – or, like that Nike ad, 'Just do it'. Once you begin you will be amazed at the results.

BREAK-FAST Like a KING

You are about to discover:

What to eat and when, in order to maximise overall health, well-being and weight loss

How to establish a routine for chewing your food

The importance of eating a large breakfast

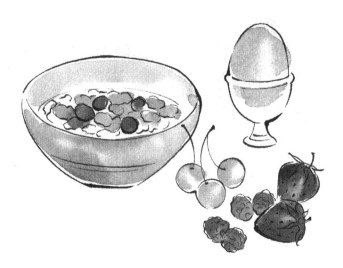

Today's Menu

Breakfast
Green tea, oat porridge with fresh fruit and linseed oil, and spelt bread with avocado spread (see page 242)

Lunch
Vegetable risotto with olives, basil and Parmesan (see page 243)

Dinner
Rice burgers with beetroot ragout and asparagus (see page 244)

Today you'll be eating a big breakfast, something that you'll need to do every day of the Viva Mayr Diet and, if you want to maintain its dramatic benefits, for the rest of your life. In fact, it's time to get used to starting big and becoming progressively stingier with your meals as the day goes on.

When I was in my early twenties, I went on a diet that I continued for several months. It made absolutely no difference at all to my weight. It wasn't what you would call an overly sophisticated diet; basically, it consisted of missing breakfast. I would get up, drink a cup of tea and go to the office on an empty stomach. The first thing I ate would be a cheese and coleslaw sandwich for my lunch. Still, my tummy and thighs remained the same size. I couldn't understand it. How could I skip a whole meal and not lose any weight?

According to Dr Stossier, what I should have been doing

was skipping dinner instead of breakfast. The old adage 'breakfast like a king, lunch like a prince and dine like a pauper' is at the heart of the Viva Mayr philosophy.

Like everything else in life, our digestive system has a rhythm. Biological rhythms are what enable us to live as long as we do. Through these rhythms cells regenerate, which increases our life span. In fact, humans are able to live to such a ripe old age *because of* the rhythmical nature of our body processes. Our life may be finite, but nature works to keep us young and healthy by adaptation and positive selection on just about every level, including cellular and molecular. Healthy molecules, for example, vibrate rhythmically. Old, unhealthy ones lose this ability and our bodies automatically dismantle and replace them. It is a form of self-healing that means we can keep going on … and on.

We regenerate when we sleep, so that in the morning we are full of energy and ready to tackle an action-packed day. And just like our bodies, our digestive systems are at their most active in the morning.

'We don't have the same digestive capacity for 24 hours,' said Dr Stossier. 'Just as our bodies and minds tire towards the evening, so does our digestive system. In the morning we can digest basically anything at all. This is the time to eat a lot and it is also the time to eat raw foods, which are more difficult to digest.'

If you want to lose weight, you need to be aware of your digestive system's rhythms and eat accordingly. So I had it all the wrong way round. Instead of skipping breakfast, I should have been starting the day with my biggest meal and then significantly reducing the amount of food I ate towards the end of the day. But please don't do what a friend of mine did: she ate a huge breakfast, and still ate the same big lunch and dinner she always had.

'This Viva Mayr thingy doesn't work,' she told me, after four weeks of eating like a lunatic.

Funny that.

To adopt the Viva Mayr approach to health, you need to stop thinking of breakfast as a time to throw something down your throat before rushing off to work and getting on with the rest of the day. Really make the time to turn breakfast into something serious. Forget about sticking to a traditional bowl of cereal. By all means eat some cereal, but also take advantage of your strong digestive system to eat raw foods. So add fruit to your cereal – lots of it. Or eat some fruit beforehand.

Today you're going to start breakfasting like a king. The important thing to bear in mind is that you can eat anything you want at breakfast. Nowadays I always make sure I have something raw at breakfast, even if it's just a few grapes or an apple or some juice. Of course, breakfast coincides with the time when you are rushing to get the kids to school and yourself to work so, practically speaking, it's not the ideal time to sit around eating. In fact, most of us are lucky if we manage to stuff in a Weetabix before heading off to get on with our day. But if you're going to adopt the Viva Mayr approach, then you may have to get up a little earlier. If that sounds daunting, read on. As you will learn in the next chapter, late dinners should become a thing of the past, which has the knock-on effect of making you far more energetic first thing in the morning.

Wake up and chew

Your morning routine will become increasingly important. Try this today and aim to keep to it strictly for the remainder of the 14 days. By then, chances are it will have become a habit. You will enjoy maintaining it as you feel your body respond well to being fed what and when it most naturally *wants* to be fed. Imagine a pyramid – the heavy base represents the quantity of food that you'll begin with every morning, narrowing as it reaches the apex, which is the amount you'll be eating for dinner.

I can hear you having an 'I have nothing to wear' moment. *What on earth do I eat?* I can hear you asking. *And where do I begin?*

Very simply, begin, as always, with a cup of hot or warm water. While you are sipping this, do your morning stretches and contemplate the day ahead. You are going to totally overhaul the way you have been eating up until now. Not only are you going to carry on chewing, but you're also going to learn to breakfast like a king.

At the back of the book, you'll find recipes for the first 14 days' menus and some additional Viva Mayr specialities, so every day you will be able to choose a good breakfast. If what's on today's menu doesn't appeal, you can certainly choose something else, but I'd like you to bear with me and try what's on offer. Today I'd like you to begin by eating something you may never have considered for breakfast – just to get you used to changing your habits. We are going to eat raw tomato and avocado with linseed oil and some seeds sprinkled on top. It may seem an unlikely breakfast, but it's ideal. What's more it's a perfect accompaniment to a delicious omelette, which will give you a great start to your day. Slice the avocado and drizzle about a teaspoon of linseed oil over it. You can layer it on top of a slice or two of wholemeal, spelt or rye bread, if you wish, or eat it with bitefuls of your omelette. You can sprinkle salt and pepper on your avocado and tomato if you want to. Sea salt is preferable for its mineral content.

If you don't fancy avocado and tomato, then go for something else. If it seems too odd for you to eat vegetables first thing then go for some muesli, but make sure it's served with some fruit. Or you could opt for a Spanish option – rubbing olive oil, tomato and garlic into some lightly toasted bread. Or how about some crudités? Cut up carrots, celery, cucumber – or whatever you feel like – and dip them into a delicious spread, such as the clinic's herbal spread (see page 279).

Above all, remember to chew, chew and chew again.

A little refreshment

You will also need to get into the habit of drinking teas that will support your digestive system, and help to set you up for the day ahead. Here is a list of suggestions. If you have other favourites, by all means drink them. And don't forget to check out the recipes on pages 275–7 as well.

Green Tea Activates your blood circulation, reduces blood pressure, increases concentration, invigorates and revitalises.

Rosemary Tea Improves the circulation of the brain, helps concentration, activates your metabolism; see page 92 for the recipe.

Liver Tea Encourages healthy liver function and regeneration. Note: this undoubtedly tastes bitter, but it's worth remembering that *anything* bitter supports the liver. Avoid brewing for too long, or it may become unpalatable. Try to drink at least one cup a day during the 14-day programme. To prepare liver tea, add a teaspoonful each of yarrow, wormwood and dried berberis (barberry) bark to boiling water and follow the instructions on page 275.

Yarrow Tea Encourages the metabolic functions of the liver, helps to prevent headaches, migraine and vertigo, and eases liver, gall bladder, stomach and gut complaints. Note: this isn't as bitter as liver tea, but it may still be an acquired taste; see page 275 for the recipe.

Fresh Ginger Tea Encourages healthy digestion, eases digestive complaints (including nausea) and arthritis, and encourages good circulation. Note: this is my personal favourite; see page 275 for the recipe.

How to prepare your teas

For one cup of tea, take a teabag or a pinch of dried herbs and place them in the bottom of your cup. Add very hot water and steep for 30 to 60 seconds (except ginger tea; see page 275). On the Viva Mayr Diet you'll be drinking tea for its hydrating effects rather than the therapeutic qualities of the herbs they contain. If you prepare your teas in this way, they are the ideal alkaline liquids (see page 00), which will support your digestion and metabolism.

Juice and water shouldn't be drunk with meals, as they can dilute the digestive enzymes and make them less efficient. You can, however, have a little herbal tea with your breakfast, but drink it by the teaspoonful, and take only a little. Throughout the day, you can drink anything you like between meals, including milk, herbal teas, water and fruit or vegetable juices. Tea and coffee are off the menu because of the caffeine they contain, as are fizzy drinks, but you can choose from all of the other alternatives to make sure you stay hydrated. Water is most definitely your best bet (see page 133).

Respect your body clock

We need to pay attention to the way our bodies work to get the most out of them. To stay healthy, we have to respect what suits our bodies and when. Our body clocks are rather like the seasons – part of a natural order we cannot change. They are essential to our health and longevity. Our body clocks are essential not only for the renewal of healthy cells and processes, but also for the elimination of what is old and diseased. Without this renewal and regeneration, we would age very quickly. And although we cannot prevent ageing, the lifestyle we choose can control *how* we age. When we support our natural body clock – by eating in harmony with it, for example – we also support our natural ability to heal, which in turn helps to slow down the ageing process.

For the next 14 days (and preferably beyond) make a commitment to eat fruit or vegetables – or both – for breakfast. According to our body clock, this is the ideal time for digestion, so, ultimately, the best time to fit in foods that take a little more work to digest. If you can't bear the thought of raw carrots early in the morning, then how about investing in a juicer and making carrot and mango juice? There are lots of variations, such as lemon, pear and cucumber; red pepper, carrot and orange; papaya and celery blended with a little mint; or a handful of berries with apple and celery. Anything goes, as long as it's fresh – and raw. Juices are a great way to 'eat' fruit and vegetables, as part of the process of digestion has already been done for you.

How do you feel after your large breakfast? As though you've eaten too much? That feeling will soon pass. You are going to start eating less in the evening, from Day Eight onwards, so in future you will be hungrier first thing in the morning.

Make breakfast your favourite meal

At the Viva Mayr Clinic, breakfast is the highlight of the day. Well, the biggest highlight before lunch, that is. The first morning I was there I was greeted with the news that I was allowed two items, not just one, from the menu. And that is alongside the mainstay of spelt bread and my daily dose of oil (see page 43–4), as well!

At first I was so over-excited I could barely choose. Finally I opted for the herb spread (see page 279 for the recipe) and a soft-boiled egg. Never has a breakfast tasted so good. I sprinkled sea salt on my free-range egg and the flavour of the salt and the yolk really complemented each other. I think this was the first time that I have actually *tasted* an egg yolk. It was creamy and warm. I found the chewing thing much easier, too. I made an effort to take as long as I could. I was determined to finish after Annie this time.

I really thought about every mouthful. I focused on what I was eating and savoured every moment. I sipped my rosemary tea, which tasted lovely. A man from one of the adjoining tables struck up a conversation with us, and offered to lend us his *Daily Mail* (a very expensive luxury in Austria). Charming as he was, I almost wanted to tell him to shut up. Couldn't he see that I was in a zone? Poor old Annie was not allowed the spread, but she did have an egg, which made a change from potatoes. We left breakfast feeling healthy, thin and full. A great combination. Added to which we had the *Daily Mail.* What's not to like?

In summary ...

- There is reputable science behind the age-old saying, 'Breakfast like a king, lunch like a prince, dine like a pauper'.

- It is important to eat a hearty breakfast and to respect your body clock.

- Although skipping breakfast might seem like an easy way to lose weight, it really isn't.

- Your digestion is at optimal level in the morning, so this is the time to eat as many raw foods as you can.

Case Study

Elisabeth, 32, Brighton

Once I left the clinic, I knew the most difficult part of sticking to the Viva Mayr Diet would be finding the time to eat properly, especially in the morning. I was used to doing everything within a really strict time frame. I have two boys, aged seven and nine, to get ready for school, sports kit to find, packed lunches to make and a husband who enjoys a freshly made cup of tea. I am not a priority and I couldn't imagine how I would ever change that.

Now, six months later, I have managed it. We get all the school kit ready the night before. I wake up, have my cup of hot water (making tea for my husband at the same time), and start laying the table. I cut up some fruit — whatever happens to be in season — and then get the boys up and dressed. Then I cook my eggs, slice my avocado and tomato, or make my muesli — whatever I am planning to eat. Half an hour before we are due to leave, I make sure I am sitting down. I start with the fruit and then eat my main course. I take my time. My husband has got used to me doing this, so takes over the childcare until I have chewed my way through a large breakfast.

The fact is that if you really want to make time to eat, then you can. The world will not fall apart because you are too busy chewing to run around after everyone else. I have noticed that now I no longer make myself available to do every little thing for them, the boys manage quite well by themselves. As does my husband!

At the weekends, when we don't have to rush to get anywhere, I allow myself a longer time slot and eek out breakfast to 45 minutes. I really take it slowly and enjoy every moment. I can chew a blueberry for half a minute. The difference in taste is unbelievable. I don't think I really tasted food before; it is just totally different when you chew it properly. One side-effect of all of this focusing on my food is that I can no longer eat junk — it just tastes too disgusting. So my weight has stayed as low as it was when I left the clinic. I am thrilled.

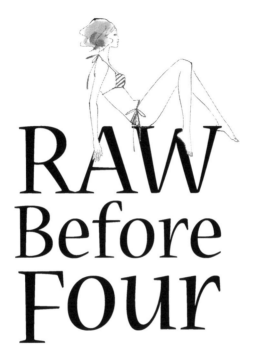

RAW
Before
Four

You are about to discover:

How to eat raw before four

Why it is so important to eat your raw foods before the magic hour of four pm

That you are well on the way to the new Viva Mayr you

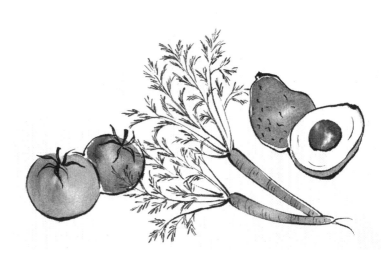

Today's Menu

Breakfast
Forest herb tea, and linseed yoghurt with papaya and maple syrup (see page 245)

Lunch
Fruity sprouted salad with linseeds, and celeriac with slices of turkey ham, vegetables and fresh herb cream (see pages 245–6)

Dinner
Asian-style vegetables with lemongrass and herbs (see page 247)

Welcome to Day Six. How are you feeling? Comfortable? Slimmer? Have your energy levels kicked in yet? If not, be patient, it's early days. If you are, you're going to keep feeling better and better.

By now you should really be getting to grips with the chewing thing and you should also be getting used to eating a hearty breakfast. And above all you should be feeling a little thinner.

Now you are ready to begin Day Six. Today you are going to take advantage of your body's capacity for digesting those essential raw foods and eat plenty of raw before four. You'll find the recipes for today's menus on pages 245 to 247, as well as some alternative suggestions, which include a scrummy sweet potato salad for lunch, as well as fillet of poached trout with lemongrass for dinner. If you like, mix and match the meals to create a combination that suits you. And don't forget to drink your lovely herbal teas as well.

The concept of eating 'raw before four' forms the basis of another crucial Viva Mayr motto. This simply means that you cannot eat *any* raw food after four pm. The reason is that your body will not be able to digest it effectively. As we learned in the previous chapter, our digestive systems are at their most effective at breakfast time. Because raw food takes more work to digest, it's the optimum time to add it to your diet. As the day goes on, our digestive capacity is reduced, and the Viva Mayr Diet is designed to accommodate that.

If this all seems a bit technical, bear with me. If you're going to believe in the Viva Mayr Diet, then you need to understand it. In a nutshell, when our digestive systems are working well, we use enzymes to digest our food. When it is not – for example, when we eat too late at night, or we eat raw food after the four pm deadline, which exhausts the digestive system – our bodies send the food we eat to our body's healthy bacteria, known as intestinal flora, to digest. This results in fermentation because the bacteria metabolise food in a different way from the enzyme approach. Our bodies create a lot of alcohol and acid in our systems, which has the same effect on our insides that alcohol has – it creates gases and even more fermentation, and it slows everything down. Long-term, this can result in something known as 'Leaky Gut Syndrome', where large spaces develop between the cells of the gut wall allowing bacteria, toxins and food to leak through into the bloodstream (see pages 159–62).

Digestion occurs with the help of our enzymes and is supported by healthy bacteria (intestinal flora). There needs to be a balance between these two, and this balance can only occur if you eat the right things at the right times. In other words, no raw food after four.

The reason why raw foods are so hard to digest is that they contain a lot of vitality, which requires a lot of energy to break down. It is fairly logical; a plant has its own life and to digest it you need to remove its identity and assimilate it into your own system; this is what digestion is. This presents much more of a challenge for your body than a cream bun would, or something that is cooked and has had its identity removed. Raw foods are vital and chock-full of energy, but it is precisely these qualities that make them such a hazard for a tired metabolism. They are also full of fibre, which makes them more difficult to digest later on when our digestive enzymes are not so plentiful. So while they are extremely good for us at the right time of day, they can play havoc with our digestion when we eat them too late.

Eat raw when your body can deal with it

Governments all across the Western world are heavily pushing the 'five-a-day' rule for fruits and vegetables. That's all very well, but they haven't made any distinction between raw and cooked. And that's as important as getting the right quantity in. Try very hard to avoid eating fresh lychees after dinner, for example, or an apple before bed. Why? Because if we eat too much raw food too late, it will sit fermenting in our intestines rather than being digested quickly and its nutrients taken up by our bodies.

Today you started with your gloriously abundant breakfast, which included at least some raw fruit and/or vegetables. Don't tell me you can't find anything fresh or that you don't have time to cut up an apple. Everyone has time to eat a satsuma in the morning, or even nibble a raw carrot. If you are pressed for time first thing, why not make a fruit salad the night before and refrigerate it until you need it? When the flavours of the fruits have mingled, it will be even more delicious. There is no need for a recipe here – just toss in what you like, including pears, apples, apricots, satsumas, mango, grapes and berries. Blanched almonds – or any other nuts and seeds – are OK, too. If you want banana you should add it just before you serve it, though, or it will go brown.

If you feel like trying some vegetables but don't want to get up early to peel them, prepare your carrot, pepper and celery batons, for example, the night before and stick them in the fridge in some cold water. They will be crisp and fresh in the morning.

Eating raw for lunch

Lunch is relatively easy, as your system is still strong enough to cope with the digestion of raw foods. Take advantage of this fact, and try to eat salads for lunch as often as you can. There is no point in wasting lunch with cooked foods. If you have no choice in the matter, then at least eat some raw carrot batons, an apple, or something uncooked. Although your system can cope with raw food at this time of day, it will not like it if you wolf it down practically whole. Salad is the thing to have for lunch. Today, go for the delicious vegetable salad (see page 230 for the recipe). If you are heading to the office, then pop the salad in a box and take it with you. Remember as always to chew and to take your time. Really savour the flavours. Cut your food into little pieces. Time your lunch so you make sure you take half an hour to eat it.

Even if you don't follow the Viva Mayr menu plans strictly, it is crucial both during the diet – and for the rest of your life – to avoid eating raw foods after four. This rule applies to all fruits and vegetables. Other foods, such as meat, fish, nuts and seeds can be eaten after four, but preferably not after six pm! Confused? Read on; it will all make sense shortly!

Autointoxification
(Or, *Why you should only eat raw before four*, by Dr S)

Imagine the intestine is like a long tube from your lips to your bottom. The surface of this intestine is a membrane, which means that all the processes in the intestine (digestion) can take place without influencing our body's other delicate processes. The lining of the intestine is efficient and essential. There are literally billions of bacteria in our intestines that support the digestive process, but they cannot be allowed to go through the mucous membranes and enter our bloodstreams. If only one bacterium passed through, our immune system would be immediately activated to 'kill it'.

When we eat raw food after four (this is a rough time, not set in stone, but approximately when the average person's digestion becomes less efficient, as we wind down towards the end of the day), it will ferment in our intestines, because our bodies cannot effectively digest raw food after that time of day. This fermentation creates alcohol, acids and gases, and it irritates the membrane of the gut (largely because the alcohol produced dissolves the fatty membrane) and creates holes. The result? Leaky Gut Syndrome. These holes in the gut allow bacteria, acids, toxins and food particles to enter our bloodstream, where they must be dealt with by the immune system. Over time, the immune system becomes overloaded, and as these substances begin to circulate around our bodies, we see a process known as 'intestinal autointoxification', which can be extremely dangerous. See pages 159–62 for more details.

Don't blame the food

I have often heard people say that raw foods 'don't agree' with them. This is just not possible. What doesn't agree with them is the way or the time of day they are eating raw foods. It is true that solely eating raw foods does not guarantee you health. For example, our bodies find it much easier to assimilate the nutrients in some foods when they are cooked – carrots, or tomatoes, for example. Furthermore, however, and more relevantly, our bodies are probably unlikely to make use of the cornucopia of nutrients in raw vegetables simply because they are badly digested. If we eat them too late, our bodies ferment them, and turn them into acids, rather than digesting them into a form that our bodies can immediately use. So if you have the impression that raw foods don't agree with you, it isn't the food that's at fault!

There are several reasons why raw food could cause you discomfort. You are either eating them too late, or your digestion is impaired and needs to be detoxified. Dr Stossier told me a story from his childhood, which illustrates how our digestive systems can be badly affected by toxins: 'When I was a child, I often went with my grandparents, who lived in the country, to a farmer to get milk. My grandmother had a special milk jug that she thoroughly cleaned after bringing home and distributing the milk. She always made sure that the milk jug was cleaned again before being filled with fresh milk. She did this based on the knowledge and experience that even small amounts of milk remaining in the jug would turn sour very quickly. When fresh milk is added to the sour milk left over from the previous day, the fresh milk would also turn sour quickly.'

Now imagine your digestive system in place of the milk jug. If there is a fermentation process going on in there, it will affect all the new foods we eat. The bacteria will, in fact, taint everything that enters. And this is where you get flatulence or bloating after a meal. And if that flatulence smells bad, then just think about what must be going on in there. *Yuck!*

'To prevent unpleasant reactions such these, the recommendation is not to eat raw foods at all in the evening,' said Dr Stossier. 'This applies to salads, fruit juices and fruit. Cooking such foods – for example gently and briefly boiling, braising or steaming them – significantly improves digestibility and our ability to handle such foods. Therefore, this recommendation does not represent a significant restriction or risk vitamin deficiency. Instead, it leads to greater vitality and health.'

Putting it into practice

Since being at the clinic I have tried to avoid eating raw food after four, as much as possible. This is particularly difficult now, as I often come home late from work to find my husband has ordered a take-way.

A few days ago, I had no choice but to eat late – and raw. I ate some tabouleh salad with hummous and Arabic bread, normally something I would digest without difficulty, but it was almost 10pm and as I was eating I realised what a bad idea it was. I was so hungry I just couldn't stop myself but my new 'Viva Mayr' trained body soon went into shock. I can't tell you how badly I slept! My body seemed almost to be fighting a fever. I kept waking up in a sweat and was really uncomfortable. If I was faced with a similar situation again, I would do as Dr S suggests and simply not eat at all.

In summary …

- It is extremely important to avoid raw foods in the evenings.

- We should all stock up on raw foods during the day (before four pm), to get the nutrients we need.

- The fermentation process caused by eating raw foods too late in the day causes all sorts of digestive problems, potentially leading to Leaky Gut Syndrome.

Case Study

Karen, 58, Harrogate

I spent most of my life eating toast and marmalade for breakfast. It never occurred to me to eat anything else until I discovered Viva Mayr and thought about how I was going to furnish my body with enough raw food to stay healthy. Suddenly I had to think about eating something raw first thing, and the idea did not appeal! I couldn't give up my toast, melting butter and homemade marmalade, so I made a few adjustments. I began by eating something raw first. The least painful raw food I could manage was seedless grapes. On other occasions, I went for half a grapefruit or some apple slices. Then I had my toast and marmalade. I don't want to sound like the school prefect, but after a few weeks of eating fruit first thing, it became a habit and it's now as hard to break as my toast and marmalade one. Actually, if you asked me to give one up, I'm not sure which one it would be any more.

STOP when you're FULL

You are about to discover:

How to stop eating when you are full

How to eat smaller portions

How to avoid the pitfalls that people often fall into when dieting

An achievable morning routine that gets your day started the right way

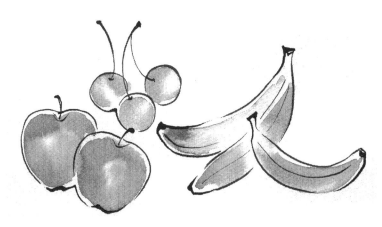

Today's Menu

Breakfast
Green tea, and hummus with vegetables sticks (see page 248)

Lunch
Rocket salad with smoked salmon and horseradish, and buck-wheat crepes with parsnips and chervil cream (see page 249)

Dinner
Tarragon tofu burgers with fresh vegetables stew (see page 251)

Y ou could be forgiven for believing, even today, that you should finish what's on your plate. After all, you are a well-brought-up person who probably spent your childhood being told to 'eat up', and being regaled with stories about starving Africans. In fact, I regularly find myself telling my children to finish their meals. During the Second World War, a whole generation was encouraged to eat whatever was on their plates. And, in some cultures, swathes of the population don't know when or what they will eat next. It's not surprising that we have been force-fed the idea that we need to clear everything from our plates, or we will be creating waste. Things are now different here in the West, where we almost always have enough (and, in most cases, more than enough). So we need to change our eating habits and get to grips with the idea that not finishing everything on our plates can be a *good* thing. Better still, give yourself much smaller portions to begin with, so you don't waste anything. We all have to learn to stop when we feel we've had enough. Even slightly before.

But how exactly do you know when you've had enough?

'If you eat slowly and chew well, you will know when it is enough,' says Dr Stossier. 'It is very difficult to describe the feeling of *enough*, as it is different for everyone. One thing is for sure: when button pops off your jeans, it's too much.'

You need to learn to listen to your body rather than looking at what is on your plate. Again, it's a question of training – just as you trained yourself to learn to chew. The secret is that when you feel full, you've eaten a bit too much. Therefore, next time eat a little less and see how you feel. Try to recognise the difference between actual hunger and habit. We often crave food just because we see it rather than because we are truly hungry. We also sit down to meals when we aren't actually hungry, because we are creatures of habit.

I discovered by accident that I was eating much more than I needed. One day, when I was in the middle of lunch, I had eaten half an omelette and some green beans when I had to take a work call. I left the table (Dr S would have been angry with me for allowing work to interrupt my lunch, but there are some things you can't avoid) to take the call that lasted about half an hour. By the time I came back to my lunch, it looked extremely unappetising. But I also noticed that I just wasn't hungry anymore. My brain had clearly told my stomach that lunch was over, and it was time to digest.

Now I give myself between half and a third of what I used to eat. For example, instead of having two pieces of toast with my boiled egg for breakfast, which I have always thought was what I needed to get me through to lunch, I have one. And I chew it *incredibly* slowly. Part of the reason why I find this so easy could, of course, be linked to the fact that the new Viva Mayr me always starts the day with fruit – so maybe I'm just not that hungry by the time I get to my toast. But you get the idea. Cut down on your portions by a quarter or even a half. You will still live to see your next meal, I promise.

If you are struggling to know when you've had enough, stop yourself, say five minutes before you would normally finish – or when there is about a quarter of your usual food intake still remaining on the plate. Go off and do something different for 10 minutes, and then come back and see if you are still hungry. I can promise you that you won't be. So give yourself a smaller portion, and ask yourself as you head towards the finish line: *Do I really need the rest of this?* If you do, eat it. If not, try the 'wander off for 10 minutes' trick.

A little training

Try to train yourself to start eating less by having just a chunk of spelt bread (let's say one or two of the 70g pieces you made) with a cup of vegetable soup for dinner. It may not sound like a substantial meal, but if you chew it extensively and take the soup with a small spoon, you will soon get that 'absolutely enough' feeling, which you will experience as a sense of well-being. I hate the feeling you get after a huge lunch, when all you want to do is go to sleep, and you have no energy to move. What I find so refreshing about eating less is that I leave the table feeling invigorated and energised, rather than soporific. If you eat the optimum amount at mealtimes, then the food will actually give you energy as opposed to sapping it, as your body struggles to cope with digesting the enormous amounts of scoff you have just eaten.

Tricks to keep you on the wagon

It takes only a few days of eating less to get a feeling of having had enough. Here are some other tricks to help you along and to stop you from falling off the wagon:

- Use a smaller plate. For example, choose a plate for your main meal that you would normally use for a piece of toast – in other words, a 'starter-sized' or side plate. It is amazing how psychological eating is, and how just using a smaller plate will reduce the amount you eat. As simplistic as it sounds, your brain will tell your well-trained stomach that 'you have finished your plate, therefore you have had enough'.

- Make sure you drink a lot of water between meals, to ensure you don't mistake thirst for hunger pangs.

- Take your time. The longer you take over a meal, the more likely your brain is to send messages to your stomach saying you have had enough. It's a psychological benefit of eating slowly.

- Try to eat a small meal of just soup and spelt bread for dinner at least twice a week and you will get used to eating less. Some evenings, when I get home from work too late to eat, I just have a glass of red wine and eat some almonds. Then I wake up hungry and ready to breakfast like a king.

- Sleep well. This will happen naturally if you don't eat late at night. Tiredness leads to cravings for high-energy foods.

- Exercise every day, even if it's only pushing your children on a swing, walking instead of taking the car or bus, doing some physically demanding housework, or running up and down some stairs (see pages 82–3). Take every opportunity you can to move.

- Remember that eating junk food will not give you that 'I've had enough' feeling because it doesn't contain any nutrients. Your body will still be craving the nutrients it needs.

The right-sized portion

The good news is that Viva Mayr isn't worried about your portion size, and you can, actually, eat as much or as little as you want. The idea is that when you begin to chew properly and eat the right types of foods, you will feel full sooner and will naturally reduce your portion sizes until they are just right for you – no matter how mammoth they were to begin with. In fact, you'll find that after even just a week on the Viva Mayr Diet, you'll be aghast at the size of the portions offered in restaurants, for example. You'll wonder how you could ever manage to eat all that food.

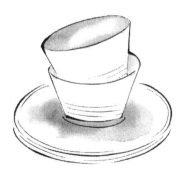

Avoiding the pitfalls

Don't get discouraged; you are changing the way you live and eat, so it is going to be tricky at times – but keep at it.

Remember there is no need to go hungry – drink a glass of water or eat some almonds. And no, you do not *need* that Krispy Kreme.

Don't despair if you can't cook one of the meals suggested – just use your common sense. The meal suggestions are there as a support not to stress you out so if you would like to eat something else then do, as long as it is within the parameters of the diet (no raw after four and so forth).

If you feel it's all too much to remember please don't just decide to re-member nothing at all – take it one thing at a time, go back to the first chapter and read it again, inwardly digest (I can't resist this pun) all the different points.

How are you feeling?

So how are you feeling? Healthier and thinner, I hope. After seven days of the Viva Mayr way, you should really be starting to feel the benefits. Take out the list of aims you wrote down at the beginning of the week. Do you feel that you have achieved any of them? If you haven't fully achieved them, do you feel that you are on your way? Maybe you are not even close yet, but let's look at some of the things you have undoubtedly achieved so far:

- You know what kinds of food you should be eating to ensure a long, healthy and slim life.

- You know how to cook them.

- You know what foods you should be eating at what times of day to maximise the nutritional benefits and minimise digestive difficulties.

- You know how to exercise effectively, and you should already be feeling the benefits of moving.

- You know how to chew your food properly, in the way it was intended to be chewed, and in a way that will ensure you stay healthy, slim and free from digestive problems.

- As you will see on Day Ten, all this knowledge will mean that you now have a better chance of avoiding life-threatening diseases, such as diabetes and cancer.

And …

- You can make spelt bread (and not a lot of people can say that!).

Assess your own progress by asking yourself the following questions …

1 If someone were to offer you a Krispy Kreme doughnut now, would you eat it?

2 Can you watch someone wolfing down their food without wanting to go over and tell them to slow down?

3 Are you ready for the next seven days of the Viva Mayr Diet?

If you only answered 'yes' to the last question, then you are an A-grade student. If you answered 'yes' to two of them, you get a B; three, and you're in the Cs. But that's no reason to give up. There is a lot more to learn in the next seven days of the Viva Mayr Diet. You will learn when, what and how much to drink. You will learn how to avoid a bloated stomach forever. You will learn how the Viva Mayr Diet can keep you young looking.

Let's get on with Day Eight...

Diet for life

Don't think of Viva Mayr as a diet. Although you will be making broad-scale changes to what and when you eat, you are, ultimately, making a life change, a life choice as well. You have taken a great big step towards a slimmer, healthier you. The Viva Mayr Diet is not a chore to be borne for two weeks, like some other diets; rather, it is a way to radically overhaul the way you look and feel by incorporating some small changes. Eating earlier, avoiding raw food after four, chewing efficiently and for longer, are massively easy changes to make, and they really will produce dramatic results. You can more or less eat anything you like, as long as you eat it slowly, in the right volume, and at the right time of day. In fact, the Viva Mayr Diet is every woman's dream diet. You eat food, all sorts of food, that makes you look and feel great. You take time to eat, to relax, to enjoy your food and you can even drink wine. This is not a diet, it's a gift!

In summary …

It's important to listen to your body, and learn to recognise the signals telling you that you've had enough.

Use some of the many tricks outlined here to teach yourself only to eat until you've had enough.

Recognising dieting pitfalls can help you to avoid them in future.

Case Study

Maureen, 33, Sheffield

I used to think it was rude not to finish my food, so even if I knew I was full, I would keep going. I think it was my upbringing! The fact that I didn't actually have to eat everything on my plate now that I am over the age of consent came as a bit of a revelation to me! This little epiphany occurred when I was having lunch with a friend, and I was complaining that I was full but still eating. She asked me *why* I was still eating, and I suddenly thought: *It's because I can hear my mum's voice telling me to finish.* Much as I love my mum, there is no need to obey her on everything! So, from that day I stopped eating when I felt full – and not when my plate was empty. I soon realised that I had been over-eating for years. I started to lose weight, and also to crave fewer foods. Just as eating more and getting depressed because you're getting fatter is a vicious cycle, eating less and losing weight obviously go hand in hand, too.

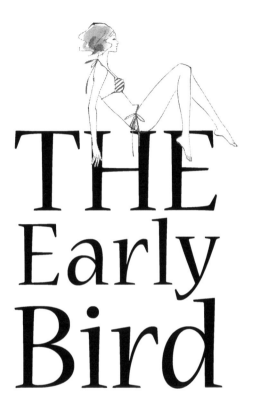

THE
Early
Bird

You are about to discover:

Why it's much healthier to eat early in the evening

The tips and tricks you need to arrange earlier meals

How to limit the damage if you do have to eat later

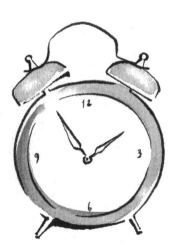

Today's Menu

Breakfast
Rosemary tea, spelt bread, and avocado, tomato and mozzarella with basil pesto (see page 252)

Lunch
Carrot and ginger soup, and turkey and rosemary skewers with sautéed fennel and courgettes, and truffle oil (see pages 252–3)

Dinner
Potato cakes with cottage cheese and linseed oil (see page 254)

You already know that raw food is off the menu in the evenings; that is, however, just the tip of the iceberg. Dr Stossier also recommends that we all eat early in the evening, ideally before six pm. We have dealt with breakfast and lunch; it's now time to look at dinner.

Of the three, this is going to be the most difficult but, at the same time, the most important change you make. There are many mistakes we consistently make when choosing and timing our evening meals, and this is something that Viva Mayr can set right once and for all.

In our culture, the main event of the day tends to be dinner. We look forward to it, we relax and unwind over the evening meal, and we take the time to enjoy other people's company. How anti-social is eating before six pm? Most of us don't even get home by then!

But Dr S is adamant that eating late is to be avoided as much as possible. The main reason is that the later we eat, the more tired we are, and the more difficult it is for our bodies to digest our food. So, because it can't digest efficiently, the body chooses other digestive options that create problems in the digestive system – such as using bacteria instead of enzymes to digest food.

Just the words 'meal time' suggest that *time* plays an important role in the process of eating. We have already seen the impact that our body rhythms have on our weight, health and longevity, and it follows that we need to take care to time our meals for the periods when our bodies are most efficient, and up to the job of digesting properly. According to that digestive capacity, we need to eat different foods and use different preparation methods for breakfast, lunch and dinner. And the evening meal needs to contain the most easily digestible foods because our system is tired. Soup and spelt bread are good choices, as are lightly steamed fish and vegetables, light risottos and other rice dishes, flans or omelettes, or vegetable stews.

Another reason why it's important to eat early is to ensure that we are hungry in the morning, when we should be eating our most substantial meal. According to Dr Stossier, when we eat late, our systems are still busy digesting what we've eaten the night before. In terms of weight control, one of the most important things we can do is to accept our bodies' rhythms, and eat less in the evening.

'I know we can't all change our lifestyles every day, but at least some days have a break for dinner around six pm, and then carry on with your evening,' suggests Dr Stossier. 'You need to eat as early as possible and eat foods that are as easily digestible as possible, such as lightly cooked vegetables and fish.'

He also suggests that if you work later than six, you should consider eating dinner at the office. This seems a little miserable to me; after all, dinner is when we relax and we spend time with our family and friends. Who wants to sit in the office with a sandwich? The compromise is to aim for eating early, and make sure it happens at least a few times a week; on the occasions you do eat later, there are some tips you can follow to help you digest the food (see page 129).

The key to sleeping well

Eating earlier ensures that we sleep better. When we sleep, two essential hormones are produced: melatonin and growth hormone. These both work during the night and are essential for regenerating our body cells. For both hormones to be produced, it is important that our body temperature is low. The later and the more we eat, the harder it is for our bodies to maintain their optimum temperature and regenerate properly at night. This is because the food we digest is turned into energy (nutritionists measure this in calories), which, in turn, raises the body temperature.

This is made worse by the fact that any food your body can't digest when it is tired ends up fermenting in your digestive system and creating even more heat. The result? We sweat, toss and turn, and generally don't sleep well – while our bodies struggle to regenerate. The result? We wake up tired and grumpy the next morning. And as an added bonus, when we sleep well we not only experience its regenerative, anti-ageing effects, but we will also be less likely to crave sugary foods to give us an instant energy boost during the day. Several studies have found that obesity is linked to poor sleep and fatigue.

The smaller the better

At the Viva Mayr Clinic, dinner is the lowlight of the day. Pretty much all that's on offer is vegetable broth and some stale bread (I mean spelt bread). I suppose it is in order to wean us off the habit of feasting in the evening. But, actually, it's quite nice going to bed without feeling stuffed full of food or drink – or both. During my first dinner at Viva Mayr, I do remember thinking that this must be a little bit like being in prison. Annie had her potatoes, of course, but I just had my broth and bread. Afterwards I took a cup of tea up to my room, my mind firmly set on those organic shortbread biscuits. But you know what? I just couldn't do it. I felt like a traitor. How could I look Annie or Brenda in the eye at breakfast? And, actually, who was I cheating? Myself, in the long run. So for my entire stay there I had a minimal dinner very early on, and I slept like a baby. I had weird dreams, but even the passing disco boat didn't disturb me. Compare that with going to bed half-cut and full of food. You know how badly you're going to sleep before your head hits the pillow. You just know that you're going to wake up feeling awful, and chances are you will spend the night tossing and turning. This tossing and turning is, of course, due in part to your raised body temperature, on account of the calories consumed.

Since I got back from Viva Mayr, I have carried on eating early whenever I can, and I really quite like it. I do it when my husband Rupert is away and I can just eat with the children. There's a silver lining to this approach, too, because I am not tempted to pick at their food when I am sitting down to eat my own! The first time I managed it, it was a revelation. Not only did I sleep better, but I loved the fact that at seven pm I still had the whole evening stretching ahead of me. It was as though I had gained an extra few hours every day, because dinner was no longer the focal point of the evening; it was over and done with, and I could get on with the rest of my day. But just as it was at the clinic, the main benefit for me was improved sleep. As a rule, I sleep terribly badly, and nothing has helped in the past. But the early eating seems to give my body time to settle down before the night ahead, and I invariably sleep well.

I have became so obsessed with eating early that I even went to a dinner party, and managed to (just about) stick to the rules. I have to admit I had become such a swot that the thought of not even sitting down to dinner until nine pm filled me with such horror that I didn't quite know how to deal with it. I didn't want to come across as a total bore. But I knew that if I did eat and drink like everyone else, I was bound to feel dreadful.

Actually, it was surprisingly easy to get away with eating next to nothing. Everyone else tucked into red wine and roast lamb, and I pretended to do the same. Obviously I had a glass or two of red wine. I ate the absolute minimum, and chewed every mouthful to a pulp. I woke up feeling great – which is most unusual after a dinner party.

So, try to eat early tonight. If you can't manage to eat before six, at least try for seven or seven-thirty, and then gradually work your way back to six over the coming days.

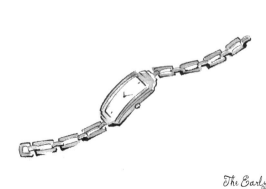

The Early Bird

Top tips to eat less at night

Book an exercise class during your usual dinner hour.

Have a big lunch, so you aren't actually hungry at dinner time.

Drink a cup of tea or a glass of water when you experience hunger.

Very slowly eat a snack such as oatcakes with cheese between six and seven pm, which will keep you going.

Plan a couple of dinners a week when you eat late with friends; view these as a treat.

Have a bath and go to bed early.

Cook light dinners and freeze them so you can easily re-heat them (not in the microwave) when you get home from work.

Arrange to go out and see a film or something that doesn't involve eating at least once a week.

If you have children and you're at home, eat with them before six pm.

Get used to overcoming the hunger barrier; it *will* pass ... once you're asleep. And imagine how much thinner you will be in the morning! If you are really desperate then eat some seeds or nuts or drink a cup of camomile tea, but honestly you will fall asleep if you don't eat – just try it!

Eating out

Going out to restaurants is, of course, tricky. You can't sit there with an empty plate! If you do go out in the evening for dinner, here's how to make the best of it. Eat *nothing* raw – and by nothing I mean not even a salad leaf decorating the plate, or a radish with the aperitif. That means no salads, and no fruit. Order something that is easy to digest, such as grilled vegetables with olive oil or a vegetable soup starter. Chew as slowly and as thoroughly as you possibly can. For the main course, opt for fish or white meat (avoiding pork, which is terribly difficult to digest) with vegetables (not salad). You could also ask for a plate of delicious cheeses and some dense bread, such as rye or pumpernickel, or wholegrain at a pinch. Your digestive system is at its weakest in the evening; you have to accept this and act accordingly. The good news is that you can most certainly have a glass of wine – or even a beer – as you go!

Maldigestion
(Or, *Why you shouldn't eat late*, by Dr S)

Maldigestion is a direct result of eating too late. Maldigestion is effectively the imbalance between our food intake and our capacity to digest it. If we eat too late, or overeat (eat too much food), we will not be able to digest it properly. As a result of this, carbohydrates that we have eaten late or in excess will be fermented in our guts instead of properly digested. When we eat too many proteins, or eat them too late, a process of putrification occurs.

When we are tired, eat late or overeat, our enzymes are unable to digest our food. As a result, this job is carried out by the healthy bacteria in our bodies, known as 'flora'. Sometimes we simply don't have enough of these healthy bacteria – for example, after a course of antibiotics, following a tummy bug, and when our diet is poor (high in refined foods and sugars in particular), which means that digestion doesn't take place as it should. Adding probiotic drinks and live yoghurt to your diet can help to redress this balance, as will eating a healthier diet.

Bacterial digestion of protein takes place through a rotting process. Yes, I know it sounds disgusting, and it is. If you don't believe me then you can reproduce this effect by allowing a piece of meat to sit out in a warm location. Over time it decomposes, and this is effectively what happens in our stomachs. So if we eat smaller quantities of protein, first and foremost our enzymes will get it all digested before this happens. Then there won't be much left for our bacterial flora to digest, so the 'rotting' will be minimal.

It has been shown conclusively that fermentation and putrification of food irritates and destroys the membrane between our intestines and our internal organs. This is the first step towards intestinal autointoxification (see page 103), as Dr Mayr called it. Put simply, this occurs when the toxins created by fermentation and putrification are reabsorbed from the intestine and trigger the immune system, causing allergies and a range of serious health problems. Once past that barrier, these toxins move towards the liver, which is our major detoxifying organ. If the liver is able to metabolise or eliminate those toxins, then great; however, this doesn't always happen. If there are too many toxins for the liver to handle, because our digestion is poor and overworked, it becomes exhausted. Furthermore, many of us put our livers under pressure by overeating fatty foods and drinking too much alcohol, and a stressed liver is unlikely to deal efficiently with the toxins created by the process of fermentation and putrification. If the liver can't deal with them, they have free access to the other organs and systems in our bodies, and will also be stored in our fat.

Does it matter if you are a night owl?

If you eat late at night – even if you are very active and awake till midnight or beyond – your digestive capacity is reduced and you will produce some toxins because of the maldigestion that occurs. As a result of this, you will begin to store water (leading to oedema, or water retention and swelling) as your body attempts to dilute the toxins to reduce their negative effects on your body's tissue. Worse still, if you retain and store water to neutralise the toxins, you will gain weight. Why? Because water retention is also weight gain.

Small and easy to digest

If you really can't make it home early enough to eat at a time that Dr Stossier would approve of, then the other option is to limit how much you eat in the evening. Invest in some oatcakes, or go for spelt bread. Try following the clinic's dinner routine, by eating some broth with a dense bread like spelt, for example. It is amazing how little you need to eat at night. It is almost as if your system knows it is not the ideal time to eat, and fills up very quickly. I do always eat something, but sometimes I am happy with just a glass of red wine, some oatcakes and a little cheese.

I remember meeting a very attractive French lady, who said that the secret to staying thin in your fifties is eating no dinner. She gave up dinner the day she turned 50, and now just has yoghurt and a Ryvita every evening. The exception to her rule is when she goes out for dinner, when she has whatever she wants. And that really is the key to success on the Viva Mayr

Diet – have a little of both, so that things don't become boring – and you don't, either! What's more, you will be amazed at how quickly you start to lose weight once you stop eating (and drinking) masses late at night.

In summary ...

- Eat as early as you possibly can, preferably no later than six pm.

- Your evening meal should be your smallest meal of the day, and contain no raw foods whatsoever.

- If you can't avoid going out to dinner, take steps to minimise the damage by eating even more slowly than usual, and as little as possible.

Case Study
Teresa, 34, Southwark

I lost six stone (38kg) over 18 months by following the Viva Mayr Diet. So, if you lose heart, read this for inspiration. Trying to juggle eating the right food, making time to eat slowly and without distractions, and eating an evening meal earlier are not the easiest things to fit around a hectic and demanding work life, not to mention a shared home. Having said that, I have made some huge and positive adjustments. Before I went to Viva Mayr, I hadn't exercised for years, ate junk food and ready meals almost exclusively, and felt pretty horrid most of the time. I'm not yet a perfect advertisement for living a Viva Mayr life, but I now have a personal trainer and work out three times a week. I eat healthy fresh food almost exclusively (and my palate has changed so much that I no longer desire what I used to eat), and I feel full of beans and happiness. It may seem a lot to take in, but it works and is worth it.

Working with my body by eating foods that are easiest for me to digest was an easy adaptation to make. Similarly, ensuring I have different oils on hand to cook with and add to food is easy, as is managing to remember to take the supplements I was recommended. I was on a strict no-sugar, no-wheat and no-fruit diet for three months, so I properly explored alternatives in the health-food aisles of the supermarket. Even though I no longer need to follow this restricted diet, I am still enjoying cooking with quinoa, and I actually prefer wheat-free pasta and muffins (no bloating), making my own soups, and so on. I now really enjoy trying new foods, too. The Viva Mayr approach to life has really helped me to make a massive lifestyle shift, as opposed to the yo-yo weight-loss and gain cycle.

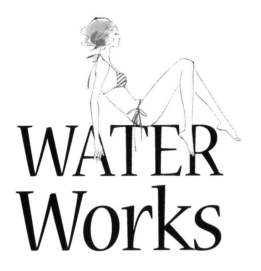

WATER
Works

You are about to discover:

Why water is so important in your daily diet

How to improve the quality of your drinking water

When to drink water, and when to avoid it

The very best water to drink

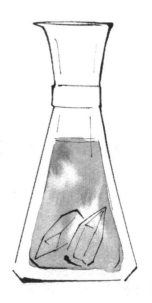

Today's Menu

Breakfast
Ginger tea, freshly pressed fruit and vegetable juice, and spelt bread with sheep's cheese (see page 255)

Lunch
Root vegetable soup, millet casserole with broccoli purée and fresh basil oil (see pages 255–6)

Dinner
Vegetable terrine with fresh herb and linseed cheese (see page 257)

Two wise old birds told me two things about water that I have tried to follow for most of my adult life. One was my grandmother, who said we should never drink during meals. She gave no reason for this apart from saying that 'it's not good for your digestion'. It was tricky advice to follow; she was Italian and an average meal spent with her could go on for about three hours. The second was my husband's grandmother, Kitty, who told me always to start the day with a cup of hot water. 'It gets your insides working,' she told me. Dr Stossier confirms that both grandmothers were absolutely right, and that there are medical reasons behind their advice.

When I first met Dr Stossier, we went out for lunch together. I was terrified. I didn't want to risk losing the opportunity to work on his book by eating or drinking the wrong thing. Imagine my relief and amazement when he ordered a risotto and a glass of wine.

'This is a man I can work with,' I thought, gleefully. The waiter asked him what water he would prefer; he deferred the question to me.

'Sparkling,' I said, happily. Big mistake. Huge. And on just about every level – as you will understand by the time you have finished reading this chapter.

Water as a nutrient

Water is one of our most important nutrients and we simply could not live without it. Some 60 per cent of our bodies are water, and we use it for dilution (of toxins, for example), transportation, regeneration and, of course, life. According to Dr Stossier, we should be drinking two to three litres of water a day, *every day*. But that doesn't mean sipping it all day long. There is a time to drink water, and a time to avoid it. It's also important that you drink the very best-quality water that you can get hold of.

So today is dedicated to water. You are already starting your day with a cup of warm or hot water. Today, you will try to ensure that you hit the two-to-three-litre target, and do so at the right times.

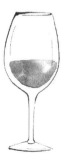

Quality water

According to Dr Stossier, drinking enough good-quality water is probably the single most important thing we can do to improve our health. Clean water has a very different effect on our bodies to polluted and toxic water. The fact that thousands of children die a day from unclean water around the world confirms this fact. Moreover, there is very good research indicating that clean, 'healthy' water can have a dramatic impact on all areas of our health and wellbeing.

Japanese researcher Emoto became famous for photographing deep-frozen water crystals under a microscope. During defrosting, a variety of crystal structures as diverse as snowflakes appeared, and Emoto discovered that these crystals were able to provide us with a great deal of information about the water, including its quality. He was able to show that the better the quality of the water, the more regular and beautiful the crystal structures.

He then subjected the water to various influences, such as music, photographs, certain words, prayers, and more, and, again and again, the water *responded to the stimuli*. These influences actually changed the water's crystal structure! Positive thoughts and prayers harmonised the crystal structure, while negative influences caused its destruction. This was the first demonstration of the fact that water takes in information and stores it. Most importantly, perhaps, it was proved that water changes its structure based on the information it holds. This sounded absurd to me, and I wasn't sure I believed any of it. That is, until I saw a man find water in my garden with the help of two sticks. Because I figured if you are able to find water with the help of two sticks then there must be more to it than meets the eye. He also told me that if you say the word 'love' to one glass of water, and 'hate' to another, you will be able to detect the difference between the two with a microscope. This I didn't fall for – but finding water with sticks, I saw with my own eyes.

Emoto discovered that the most regular crystal structures are found in fresh spring water. Water from healing springs has an even higher crystal quality. The more polluted the water, the more impurities and residues it contains, the less regular, less beautiful and less pure its water crystals. Emoto demonstrated this by taking pictures of various tap waters from large cities. Tap water is not necessarily polluted but it is not fresh and pure because it has been through so many processes. So in an ideal world we would all drink fresh spring water straight from the source. Clearly this is not possible 99.9 per cent of the time so we need to compromise.

But what has all this got to do with our digestion? If you consider the fact that water is the most important element in our body, then it makes sense that we should aim to fill our bodies with water that is full of positive influences and not negative ones. It has been scientifically proved that water has a 'memory', and therefore if the memories it contains are positive, they will have a much more beneficial effect on our overall health. Does this sound wacky? Well, it's not! Eminent French doctor Dr Jacques Benveniste found that when a substance is diluted in water, the water can carry the memory of that substance even after it has been so diluted that none of the molecules of the original substance remain. So all of those chemicals that go into our tap water, and all of the things that are supposedly 'removed' in the purification process, such as pesticides, heavy metals, hormones from human urine and pharmaceuticals, are retained there in the water's memory.

Need any more persuasion to change the type of water you drink? I thought not!

Emoto also showed how 'positivity' influences the structure of water. But 'positivity' takes place not only in our head; it also goes on in our cells and is an essential factor in healing and maintaining health. This concept is a little confusing, but I suspect it also has to do with the water's memory.

Water is the ubiquitous solvent and transport medium in the body. All metabolic processes of absorption and elimination are dependent on water, since they function best in a watery environment. Water is not only a passive reaction medium, but also an active carrier of information and so it needs to be good quality.

Which water?

Emoto's research has confirmed that the very best water we can drink is fresh from a spring. This is obviously impractical for the majority of us; however, the good news is that we can alter the water we drink to ensure that it is closer to spring water. First talk to it, in the manner that Prince Charles talks to his plants (only joking – but you really should try to stay zen and positive around your water source, even if it's only a tap).

One simple step to improve water quality is to put some stones (preferably quartz crystals, such as rose quartz, citrine, amethyst, blue quartz and jasper, which are particularly powerful cleansers) in a carafe and pour the water in on top of them. This will improve the physical quality of the water because these stones get their energy from the earth, which is then transmitted into the water. And, as we know, it remains there in the water's memory. The stones will improve the physical quality of the water by cleaning and oxygenating it, because the physical act of running it over the stones fills the water with oxygen, and the clarifying, cleansing properties of the stones make it clean.

These stones can be easily obtained from reputable suppliers (on the internet for example, on websites like www.naturalharmonycrystals.co.uk) or through the Viva Mayr Clinic (www.viva-mayr.com). They not only look beautiful in our drinking water, but they may also motivate us to drink more. Every few months, they should be rinsed well under running water and dried in the sun to restore their properties. They will last nearly forever.

Another option is to cleanse the water using less dynamic methods. One is to install filters and minerals in the plumbing of your home, which is particularly useful if the water is very hard. Dr Stossier says that water-supply pipes drain (pardon the pun) a lot of energy from the water if it has to travel a long way to get to you. That's one reason why inserting minerals, such as quartz, will help you to restore that energy.

Failing that, you can buy portable filter systems, such as filter jugs, into which you pour your water. There are also systems for 'energizing' water on the market. Some use the quartz crystals mentioned above; some use special water-processing methods, and others spin water to change its molecular make-up of the water, causing it to be energised.

Despite all the hype surrounding it, bottled water is actually best avoided – and, in particular, sparkling water. Not only does the carbon dioxide in sparkling water create gas in our digestive systems, but it is an acid substance. In fact, carbon dioxide was originally added to water to clean it!

Still bottled water is better, but bear in mind that it has probably been sitting for months inside a plastic bottle, on a shelf in some warehouse somewhere. So it's not exactly close to natural spring water. Dr Stossier calls bottled water 'a compromise'. He says, 'It is a little like a processed food – it has gone through machines. If there are no other options then drink it – if you are in a big city, for example, and the water is not good. The most important thing is to drink.'

At the Viva Mayr Clinic the tap water comes from a spring and yet they offer bottled water in the rooms. I asked Dr Stossier why this is. He told me that lots of people believe that bottled water is superior, so they have to have it on hand.

Eating and drinking do not go together

So the message so far is to drink the best water you can get your hands on, and lots of it. But you shouldn't just drink at any time. Apparently, this is where we all go wrong. The most crucial thing is not to drink when we are eating. Dr Stossier explains why: 'If we drink while we are eating we dilute our saliva just at the very moment when we need it in a concentrated form to digest our food. What you need to do is to drink water between meals. This starts the digestive process, and does not affect the digestion of your food.' The amazing thing is that many people actually only drink when they're eating. In restaurants, it would be unheard of to order food without water. But it's a habit we need to break.

Digesting food requires concentrated digestive juices. If we drink while we eat, we dilute our digestive secretions and weaken their effectiveness. As a result, our digestion suffers.

But what if you get thirsty? Dr Stossier says it is habit that makes us thirsty, and suggests, 'Try to get into the habit instead of drinking around 15 minutes before you start your meal, and then to avoid drinking water again until at least an hour after you have eaten. If you drink immediately afterwards you will again be reducing your digestive capacity.'

Only water?

Luckily we are allowed to drink small amounts of alcohol, such as wine or beer, with our meals. I love a diet that allows you to drink wine! It seems so much more realistic than a diet on which it is banned. The reason we can drink wine but not water is because wine is something you have to digest and metabolise, just like food; it is not what Dr Stossier calls a 'clear' liquid, like water, which dilutes your saliva. The bad news is Dr Stossier says we should limit our wine intake to just one glass; any more, and we start to affect our saliva, as well as our health in general.

Confusingly, alcohol is not a liquid that is required for body processes (i.e., it doesn't transport things around, or dilute them). The only substance that alcohol dissolves is fat. This is an important point, because it also digests body fat – but not in the way we'd all like, unfortunately, which explains its effect on our brain and nerve cells, which are, as we learned earlier, made predominantly of fatty acids. Even worse, our digestive system is lined with fat cells, which create its membrane, and these are also at risk of being dissolved by alcohol. We discussed the consequences of this process (in particular, fermentation, on page 103). It does so in the body, too, which explains its effect on our brain and nerves cells. Our digestive systems also contain membranes made of fat cells and are at risk of being dissolved by alcohol. We discussed the consequences of this process, especially fermentation, in the previous chapter.

So what exactly is the key difference between water and other drinks? Milk is a good example to illustrate it. Many people like to drink milk, and there are many processed milk beverages on the market. Milk is a food and not a beverage. It contains protein, carbohydrates and fats, along with a number of important minerals and, of course, some water. All of these nutrients need to be metabolised by our digestive system. In order to do so, we need our digestive system with all its qualities and strengths. When we drink foods that are not 'clear liquids', these need to be metabolised.

The same applies to fruit juices. They all contain more or less concentrated carbohydrates – namely sugar. Sugar needs to be metabolised. Fruit juices increase the risk of fermentation if we drink them at the wrong time. Soft drinks and various energy drinks belong in the same category. In addition to sugar, such beverages also contain many chemical additives that our metabolism needs to deal with.

It's all very complicated, but the basic rules are these: drink water, milk, herbal teas, and fruit and vegetables juices *between* meals, and stick to a small amount of alcohol, and perhaps a few teaspoonfuls of herbal tea *with* your meals. Even though the body has to 'digest' milk and fruit and vegetable juices as it would food, it is, says Dr Stossier, better that this is undertaken between meals so that your digestive system can concentrate on getting the maximum number of nutrients from the food you eat at mealtimes.

Starting early

If you are going to drink three litres of water a day, you need to start early, just as Rupert's grandmother suggested. Put a glass of water by your bed at night, to sip through the night and finish off in the morning, or do what I do and drink hot water instead of tea or coffee every morning. The crucial thing is to have it before you eat anything. It is a welcome drink for the intestine; it helps to activate and to cleanse your insides. Go for lukewarm water whenever possible, which is better assimilated by the body. Very hot or very cold puts pressure on it, just when you want your digestive system to be fighting fit.

If you're worried about drinking so much water that you spend all night negotiating trips to the loo, then make sure you drink two-thirds of your liquids in the morning and the remaining third during the afternoon. And, if you can't bear to drink three litres of water a day, then opt for herbal teas or vegetable broths (see page 277). The latter are also very good for quenching your appetite. Sipping water throughout the day (stopping 15 minutes before meals) is a good bet, and it will keep you well hydrated.

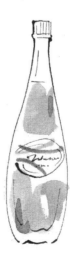

Top tips

Always drink a glass of water (preferably body temperature or warmer) first thing in the morning and last thing at night. One option is to put a glass of water by your bed at night and then drink it as soon as you wake up.

During exercise, take only a sip of water every 10 minutes or so; otherwise it interrupts your breathing. Be sure to take that sip every 10 minutes, though.

Drink as much water as you like between meals, but avoid the period 15 minutes before mealtimes, during the meal itself, and for an hour after eating.

Remember that hunger pangs can sometimes be thirst pangs. If you feel hungry between meals, try drinking a glass of water instead, or sipping a herbal tea.

Avoid fizzy water.

At work prepare a large pot of fresh herb tea in the morning, and drink it over the course of the day. You can reheat it as required, or drink it at warm temperature with a squeeze of lemon, or some fresh mint leaves.

Always travel with a small bottle of water; it will keep you hydrated, help you to maintain concentration, and stop you from getting tired.

Liquids like tea, coffee, colas, sugary and fizzy drinks contain no nutritional benefits at all and should be avoided.

Preliminary research has shown that plenty of plain water can reduce the risk of certain cancers of the colon and the urinary tract.

Herbal teas

If you prefer herbal teas, make sure they are very weak. We aren't after their therapeutic benefits (i.e., the calming effect of chamomile, or peppermint's impact on digestion), rather their taste. Steep your herbs or herbal teabags for only 30 to 60 seconds, so that you can enjoy the flavour, while benefiting from drinking a clear liquid.

Dr Stossier forgave me ordering sparkling water with my lunch, and I have since tried very hard not to drink during meals (apart from wine, obviously). I find it tough, but a good trick is to drink a couple of glasses of water just before the 15-minute cut-off point; in other words, because we shouldn't drink anything either with our meals or 15 minutes before, we can make up for it by drinking plenty prior to this. Always end the day with hot water or a weak herbal tea, such as lemon balm. You will wake up refreshed and ready for the next day.

In summary ...

- Aim for two to three litres of water each day, but think about when to drink it, and consider its quality.

- Good-quality water will encourage optimum health and well-being on all levels.

- Crystals can be used to purify and enhance the quality of your water.

- Avoid fizzy and bottled water, if you can.

Case Study

Chloe, 28, Newbury

I had never had a meal without drinking water until I had lunch with a friend who had been to the Viva Mayr Clinic. She explained in an extremely matter-of-fact way why she was drinking only a single glass of wine (and no water) with her meal. Straightaway it made sense to me. Then she explained all about water quality, and how I should avoid fizzy water – both things that I had never really considered, and which now seemed so obvious.

I have to admit that to begin with, it was really tough not drinking water with meals. I almost felt as though I had a limb missing. But I got used to it so quickly, and whenever I thought about how I was missing a glass of water, I also thought about the word 'diluting' which is what it does to your saliva and your digestive enzymes. I would immediately go off the idea of drinking. I think, though, that because I make a conscious effort to drink between meals, I actually drink more water than I did before. I really enjoy it; it is almost like a meal in itself mid-morning. I feel I am giving water its own time and place; it just seems right to me. My digestion has definitely improved and my skin is clearer. I feel more energised and have really got into a rhythm of drinking when I should. I can't believe I ever drank with food now; it seems totally alien.

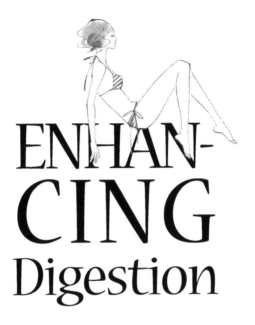

ENHAN-CING
Digestion

You are about to discover:

How good digestion is linked to good health

Why good digestion can encourage healthy ageing

Why adopting the Viva Mayr Diet can change your life – and make you even more determined to follow it

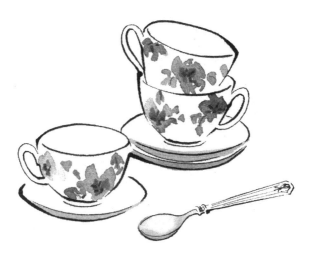

Today's Menu

Breakfast

Meadow herbs tea, and millet porridge with dried fruit and lin-seed oil (see page 258)

Lunch

Carrot and beetroot salad with fresh lemon and coriander, and lamb loin with celeriac and broccoli (see pages 258–9)

Dinner

Potato and sesame-seed patties with olive cream, courgettes and oven-roasted tomatoes (see page 260)

Ever since I was a little girl I have had a pot belly. I vividly remember standing in my stepmother's room when I was 12 years old, looking in the full-length mirror and wondering why my tummy protruded so much. I was thin everywhere else, so why the belly? It didn't seem fair. But there it was, whichever way I turned.

Until I was 32, I spent the majority of my time holding in my tummy. Then I got pregnant; what joy! Finally I could relax and let the damn thing hang out. I enjoyed it so much that I kept getting pregnant! After three children, my husband told me it was enough. The belly, of course, was worse than ever; larger and with some rather unseemly crinkly bits. Not a good look. Eventually I got so fed up with it I decided to attack it with a mild form of liposuction called Smart-Lipo. Nothing. There it was, flabby and stubborn and irritating as ever. Imagine my surprise then when Dr Stossier told me I could get rid of it in a few weeks, just by changing my eating habits.

We were in his consulting room at the clinic when he broke this news to me. He had been massaging my tummy (a daily ritual at Viva Mayr, and one I have grown quite fond of). Apparently my pot belly is not due to overeating, or excess flab, lack of sit-ups or even serial pregnancies. It is due to the fact that my small intestine is inflamed. And to protect an area that is inflamed, the body's response is to swell up. So once you remove the inflammation, the swelling goes down and you end up with a flat stomach. My belly is not flabby, it is swollen, and it is swollen to protect my intestine from further damage. Being told this was a revelation of such humongous proportions that I will never forget it.

I lay on the treatment bed and had one of those 'everything I believed before now was wrong' moments, rather like Saul on his way to Damascus. And this is the effect I want Day Ten to have on you. This is the day when you realise how crucial all of the little steps you have been taking on the Viva Mayr regime are, and why. So, sit down with a cup of hot water or herbal tea and read on.

I was stunned into silence by the news that my pot belly is not actually necessary. Dr Stossier patted it and explained, 'A lot of women have an increased amount of fat around their bellies; it is there to protect the inflamed small intestine from irritation from outside – in other words, damage to the outside of your abdomen. If you have hurt your elbow, you can simply avoid moving it; however, the only way to protect the small intestine from external damage is to put fat there. When the intestine is inflamed your body swells up to protect it from knocks and bumps, such as when you walk into a chair or someone takes a swipe at you. It is the body's defence mechanism. The fat will stay there as long as you have an irritated small intestine. No amount of dieting or sit-ups will budge it.

Once I got over the fact that I have probably done around two million sit-ups during my life in vain, I decided to try to decrease the inflammation in my small intestine to see if Dr Stossier is right. I spent 10 days at his clinic in Austria, and it was possibly the most relaxing and cleansing 10 days of my life. I admit that there were times I was so hungry I wanted to eat my lip gloss, but at the end of it I felt totally incredible. And, even better, my pot belly had almost gone. Dr Stossier predicted that the inflammation would totally vanish if I carried on for another two weeks.

Back in the real world, though, it is, of course, difficult to keep up the type of relaxing regime they offer at the clinic. But I was so inspired by the results after two weeks that I was determined to try my very best. And not just because of my formerly inflamed intestine.

I want you to do the same. By now you should be well into your Viva Mayr routine. You should be waking up with a cup of hot water, eating a hearty (and, in parts, raw) breakfast, drinking plenty of water between meals, eating a salad-based lunch, and a minimal and early dinner. Your jaw-ache should be decreasing as you get used to chewing everything 30 or 40 times. So what is all this doing for you? Not only is it keeping you thin, it is also making you *well*. Following the Viva Mayr Diet will protect you from a whole host of diseases, as well as a pot belly. Healthy people are not overweight, and because Viva Mayr ensures good health, you can and will lose excess weight, with all its side-effects.

Massage for better digestion

I have always had a soft spot for doctors and Dr Stossier in his white kit and partly matching beard inspired me with confidence. This confidence was increased when he casually pinpointed parts of my body that would hurt if poked, as a result of my dysfunctional bowels. He diagnosed this after a short examination that involved pressing my stomach and using Applied Kinesiology, which is a system in which you use muscle strength to determine the status of your body. Dr S was able to tell me what was wrong with me by pushing various limbs while placing his hand on different organs and thus working out where the weak spots were.

'You have a chronic inflammation of the small intestine,' he told me. 'And your liver is enlarged. You see the veins on your legs?'

Well, yes, now he mentioned it, I had noticed the appearance of increasingly ugly and numerous little veins all over my legs. I assumed it was because I am getting old. Not so.

'They are the result of the fermentation caused by your intestine; there is congestion being caused, resulting in the veins. Also, the redness on your face is an irritation, again caused by your intestines.'

Great, so now I could blame everything on my bowels. How has this happened?

According to Dr Stossier, it was all to do with the way I had been eating all my life. Not just the food I had been eating, but *how* I had been eating it. He said that I had been eating too fast, too late, too much and under stress; I'd also been guilty of not chewing enough. All that had to be changed, and then I would see a vast improvement in my looks, my weight, my energy levels and my sleeping patterns. Those unsightly veins might vanish, too.

Apparently my diagnosis is a common one. Almost anyone who walks into Dr Stossier's consulting room would be diagnosed with some intestinal problem.

'We have to re-train ourselves to eat in a way that our body can manage and most effectively digest,' he says. 'No one thinks about it. They just wolf their food down and expect the body to cope with it. Then they come here for an MOT, to recharge, cleanse and get their insides back to working order.'

So getting your diet right, as well as when and how you eat your food, will encourage optimum digestive health, which manifests itself as overall health and well-being. But there is also something else you can do, and this involves massage of the abdominal area – something I grew to enjoy enormously during my stay at Viva Mayr.

Do it yourself

Massaging your own abdomen is easier than you think, and it can have a very good effect on your digestive health. In some parts of the world, like Asia, for example, it is common practice to massage yourself or your friends. It's one way of getting to know and learning to respect your abdomen. What's more, it encourages a sense of well-being, by encouraging the release of endorphins (the feel-good hormones), which can help to relieve and prevent pain and discomfort, as well as lift your mood.

Nutrients are sorted and processed in the small intestine, and then channelled through the bloodstream and the lymphatic system, into the areas of the body that need them. The surface of the intestine is comprised of between 800 and 900 folds, and there are more than ten million 'villi', which are little projections that emerge from the mucous membrane lining of the intestine. These villi are important to ensure that the 'two brains' of the body (see page 65) are balanced, as they link the brain (the first brain) to the intestines (the second brain) via the vagus nerve. Therefore, massaging the intestines can not only have an immediate physical effect, encouraging better digestion and elimination, reducing constipation, and toning the muscles of the abdominal walls, but abdominal massage also enhances concentration and reduces emotional stress, as well as fatigue and depression.

There are a few things to bear in mind before you begin. The first is that you should always wait about two hours after eating, and should pay a visit to the loo to empty your bladder before you begin. Use a lotion or massage oil if you like; this is especially helpful at the beginning.

Now let's get started:

1 Start massaging from the middle of your pubic bones (the symphysis) towards your upper central abdomen (the epigastrium) with gentle, tender movements, using the palm of your hand. This massage movement follows a meridian used in acupuncture and helps to increase the energy flow in your body.

2 Now make about 50 small circular strokes in a clockwise motion around your navel. This should feel comfortable and relaxing.

3 Next widen this circular massage to include your ribcage and pelvic bones (again, repeat this about 50 times). This will benefit the large intestines.

This daily self-massage is relaxing, and is an excellent way to wake up your intestines, especially if you sometimes suffer from constipation.

When you are at the Viva Mayr Clinic, your abdomen is treated every day by a doctor using the highly beneficial Mayr abdominal treatment. This can have a positive effect on your entire digestive system, including the diaphragm, colon, small intestine, liver, pancreas and gall bladder.

I really enjoyed having my stomach massaged, especially by Dr Stossier's wife Christine. She had an extremely firm yet gentle touch and I felt she was doing a lot of good. She would get so into the massages that she shut her eyes and as my stay progressed she would comment that the state of my intestine as improving in this or that area. I felt an improvement as well. My stomach was no longer bloated and it just felt much lighter somehow, and healthier.

Now when I get nervous and feel my stomach bloating I try to emulate what she did – I just move my hand slowly around my abdomen and breathe – and it really calms me down.

The terrifying effects of obesity

Overweight isn't just unattractive; it also poses a serious risk to health on many, many levels. The good news is that sorting out your digestion can make a huge difference to your health, and one of the first signs of this is reaching your ideal weight. If you aren't someone who is overly bothered about your appearance, and can 'live with' feeling fat, then I suggest you read on!

The first effect of overweight and obesity is on your muscles and bones. Your spine will curve as it struggles to cope with the excess weight, which will lead to disc problems. In addition, your knees will weaken because they are being put under constant strain. The arch in your foot will flatten, which will irritate the musculoskeletal system, and thus irritate all of your joints and your whole spine.

Secondly, being overweight will lead to problems with your circulation. Living tissue needs nutrients and oxygen in order to survive. Without these, it does not function at optimum level. There will be extra pressure on your heart and circulation to get nutrients and oxygen to your cells. As your body mass increases, so does the need for blood and your blood pressure will automatically increase.

If you are overweight, you dramatically increase your susceptibility to metabolic diseases like diabetes. This is because there will be an increased amount of insulin stored in all that excess fat. This can result in a condition known as 'insulin resistance', because the amount of insulin we produce in the pancreas is not enough to guarantee a normal blood sugar level.

The fatter you get, the more unhealthy your eating habits are likely to become. Why? Because you will be craving saturated fats and carbohydrates in an effort to give you the energy you need to keep your whole overweight system going. In other words, the increased fat you are carrying makes you crave quick-fix foods that give you an instant energy hit (like soft drinks), but which are only going to make you even fatter. A side-effect of this is that by eating a poor diet, you will reduce your intake of vitamins, minerals and trace elements. This will also contribute to your lack of energy. And, of course, your teeth will suffer.

Calculating your BMI

Your BMI (body mass index) is based on a mathematical formula that takes into account height and weight. BMI provides a reliable indicator of fatness for most people and is used to screen for weight categories that may lead to health problems. Your BMI is the ratio of your height to your weight, and the calculations are simple:

BMI = your weight in kg divided by the square of your height in metres.

For example if your weight is 63.5 kg (10 stone) and your height is 1.68m (5ft 6in), your BMI is 63.5 ÷ 1.68 x 1.68 = 22.5

What does your BMI mean?

Under 20:	underweight
20–25	normal
25–30	overweight
30–40:	clinically obese
Over 40:	dangerously obese

If your body mass index is more than 30 you are likely to suffer from mood swings and depression, partly as a result of your inactivity because you are too depressed to actually do anything. You are likely to feel more and more on the fringes of society due to your weight, which will only add to your depression.

'Being fat is a disease,' says Dr Stossier. 'It is a medical condition, but normally you don't need pills to cure it. The cure is simply to eat less in the right way, and to exercise more.'

If you follow the Viva Mayr Diet it is physically impossible for you to become obese. Quite apart from the fact that you will be eating healthily, one of the major causes of obesity is poor digestion. And for you, that is a thing of the past.

Leaky guts

Another effect of eating the wrong way is the so-called leaky-gut syndrome I mentioned on pages 159–62. This is a result of acid built up by bad digestion, which creates holes in your intestines, allowing the toxins to pass into your bloodstream. This is one of Dr S's pet hates. He talks a lot about 'fermentation and putrification' – basically rotting food and toxic overloads – and their detrimental effect on us. Leaky gut is one of the most serious and common results of bad digestion and affects millions of people worldwide.

If you consider that 70 per cent of our immune system is located around our digestive system, you will realise how crucial good digestion is. If the small intestine is healthy (unlike mine), then it works like a selective sieve, allowing only nutrients and digested fats, proteins and carbohydrates into the bloodstream. On the other hand, if you have a leaky, unhealthy gut, then the toxins in the digestive system seep into the bloodstream. And that's where problems start. As the toxic leak becomes more serious it reaches the liver, which can be extremely serious, because it puts it under enormous pressure, causing allergic reactions throughout the body.

As soon as Dr Stossier told me about leaky gut syndrome, I was convinced I had it. I decided to do some research and come across a website called www.leakygut.co.uk. They provide a list of symptoms that will tell you whether or not you suffer from it, including:

- Abdominal pain (chronic, including spasms).

- Insomnia.

- Bloating.

- Excessive flatulence.

- Shortness of breath.

- Anxiety.

- Fevers of unknown origin.

- Haemorrhoids.

- Heartburn.

- Migraines.

- Muscle cramps.

- Muscle pain.

- Mood swings.

- Poor exercise tolerance.

- Poor immunity.

- Poor memory.

- Recurrent bladder infections.

- Recurrent vaginal infections.

- Recurrent skin rashes.

- Brittle nails.

- Hair loss.

- Swollen lymph glands.

- Food allergies.

- Constipation.

- Diarrhoea.

- Constant hunger pains.

- Depleted appetite.

- Sluggishness.

- Depression.

- Chronic fatigue.

I think I have had just about every one of these, except possibly depleted appetite. Although I do wonder how it is possible to be constipated and have diarrhoea at the same time – or to suffer from constant hunger pains but have a depleted appetite. I'll assume that not everyone suffers from *all* of the symptoms!

On the same website there is a list of tests that can be undertaken to see if you have leaky gut syndrome. My advice is this – just take it as read that you do and spend your time rectifying it as opposed to testing for it. Eat the Viva Mayr way and it will heal within weeks.

The Viva Mayr Philosophy

The Viva Mayr philosophy is that good digestion equals good health on just about every level. The goal of healthy nutrition is to prevent illnesses, such as heart and circulatory disorders, as well as metabolic disorders such as diabetes and gout, along with chronic allergies and obesity. In fact Dr S maintains that almost every modern disease can be linked to poor digestion.

Turning back the clock

One very modern disease we can at least stave off by eating well is ageing. OK, so maybe calling ageing a disease is a little radical but the scary speed with which some people age do make you wonder what they've picked up. *Eating the Viva Mayr way will mean fewer wrinkles.* Yes, you heard me correctly. If you do what Dr S tells you, you will not only feel younger, you will look younger too. I have now been eating the Viva Mayr way for five months. I saw someone I hadn't seen for a year the other day, and she told me she wouldn't have recognised me if it hadn't been for my smile.

'You look so young! What have you done?' she demanded. I think she assumed that as the author of the anti-ageing book

To Hell in High Heels, I had gone down the plastic-surgery route. I have not. It is true I did think about it, and I spent a lot of time while writing the book doing everything but having a face-lift, but since then all I have done is wear sunscreen every day and eat the Viva Mayr way.

The reason our skin responds well to the Viva Mayr diet is that the diet significantly reduces excess acidity. Our face is a good mirror of our health, and responds very quickly to excess acidity. Skin is joined to connective tissue. This connective tissue contains fibres that give our skin elasticity, vitality and suppleness – in short, everything young skin has. At the same time, however, our connective tissue is also our 'rubbish dump', and most toxins that end up there are acids. They are (temporarily) stored in our connective tissue. Because they are acids, they irritate healthy tissue, which leads to decreased elasticity and skin tone. In turn, this leaves our skin feeling 'tight' and makes it more prone to wrinkling. And so we age prematurely.

Of course we all age, but if our metabolism is overly acidic, this ageing process accelerates and intensifies. Our nails and hair, which are closely connected with our skin, are subject to a similar process. They become less elastic, our hair loses its sheen, and our nails become brittle or develop white spots.

Acid deposits in our connective tissue may also cause uncomfortable swelling, fluid deposits and muscle tension. Initially, these may be treated with massage or heat application, but in later stages, they remain permanent, because our metabolism loses its ability to compensate. Step by step, this disorder extends to larger areas of the body, causing muscles to shorten and stiffen, and impacting on our overall mobility.

Our initial response to such symptoms may be 'I am getting old'. A more appropriate response would be 'I am turning sour (acidic)', because it is possible to age without suffering from acidosis and to maintain one's vitality well into advanced age. All beings on this planet are subject to ageing. Our life is finite, but nature still attempts to keep us healthy and young through adaptation and selection in a positive sense. It is all about listening to and living by our body's clock (see page 93), which is why it is so important to eat according to those rhythms.

Live to the rhythm

Rhythms are how we renew our body tissue or cells. Individual cells have a limited life span, from a few days to years. Amazingly, our bodies have the ability to completely renew themselves (it takes about seven years in total!). Nature selects for health by recognising what is unhealthy, functionally impaired or old and removes it. In order for this health selection process to maintain our vitality, we need to maintain a functional and 'natural' level of activity and stress.

Rhythms are important and essential not only for the recognition and selection of what is healthy, but also for the elimination of what is old and diseased. Without these rhythms, we would age rapidly as a result of external (environmental) and inner (metabolic) factors and would not have a life expectancy of almost 80 years, as is common today in the Western world.

Yet, even these mechanisms cannot prevent ageing. Our behaviour can, however, control how we age. When we support our natural rhythms through weekly or daily regeneration, we support our natural healing principles.

At our initial consultation, Dr S diagnosed me as exhausted. He suggested I make sure I always have an hour a day to myself, a day a week to myself and four weeks a year to myself. I have tried to stick to this since leaving the clinic but of course it is practically impossible with a job and three children! However I do yoga three times a week if I can and this is 'my' time; just walking can be a great release too. Basically Dr S suggests you do anything – be it read a book or go for a walk or even bake a cake – that relaxes you and gives your system a chance to regenerate.

Paying attention to our natural rhythms and biological requirements is part of staying healthy. Even though such rhythms appear to be only indirectly connected with nutrition, in fact, nutrition directly impacts our natural rhythms. That's why everything you have learned so far is so crucial; not only in terms of weight loss, but the impact on how well you age for years to come.

In summary …

- Good digestion not only helps you to stay slim, but helps to avoid a number of unpleasant illnesses.

- Many of the factors affecting the speed at which we age can be controlled through a healthy diet and optimal digestion.

- The Viva Mayr Diet will not only help to prevent and treat obesity, but ensure that you reach and maintain a healthy weight.

- A pot belly is not the result of overeating, but an inflamed small intestine.

Case Study

Annie, 39, London

I went to the Viva Mayr Clinic because I was fed up with feeling below par, and had heard they did magical things. I suspected that I had some kind of food allergy, and wasn't at all surprised when Dr S told me I had candida. Candida is one of those irritating things that can affect you in so many ways; I had everything from cystitis and migraines to weight gain and tiredness, as well as bloating. It was awful. I tried a few exclusion diets at home, not eating yeast and dairy for example, but nothing seemed to work. I decided I needed more professional help.

Dr S didn't take more than a few minutes to spot that I had candida. My symptoms were pretty classic, and he uses this rather sophisticated Applied Kinesiology method of diagnosis. That was the good news. Then I was put on the Candida diet. Candida feeds on sugars, simple carbohydrates and fermented products like alcohol. It is a yeast that grows as a result of an intestinal imbalance. This can be caused by too many antibiotics, for example.

To get rid of it you have to starve the yeast for up to four weeks, which basically means eating nothing that it can feed on. So I was put on a strict potatoes-and-not-much-else diet. I won't pretend that I didn't lose the will to live after five days on nothing but boiled spuds, but the results have been incredible. I feel energised, my skin is glowing, and I am well on the way to banishing this thing from my body altogether. Now, a month later, I have been able to re-introduce most other foods into my diet and I can't tell you how good they taste. I always appreciate a simple cherry tomato now.

Not only do I feel much better, but this experience has taught me how big an effect what we eat has on our bodies. We can basically dictate how we feel by what we eat. I found the diet hard to keep up with once I left the clinic; I never wanted to see another potato! But I have stuck with the basic principles of it.

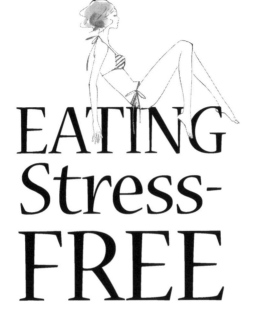

EATING
Stress-
FREE

You are about to discover:

How eating stress-free can help you to remain healthy and slim

How to avoid eating in a stressful environment

That poor eating habits are a significant stress factor

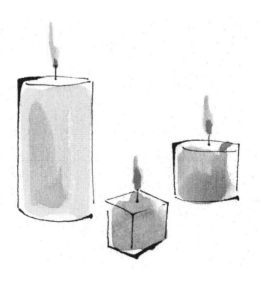

Today's Menu

Breakfast
Malt coffee, spelt bread, and Mexican omelette with fresh herbs (see page 262)

Lunch
Bowl of fresh salad, and amaranth and vegetable curry (see pages 262–3)

Dinner
Potato blinis with vegetable purée and char caviar (see page 264)

Today is all about stress – or, rather, the lack of it! Now it's time to put together all of the things you have worked on during the Viva Mayr programme, and add another essential element: eating in a stress-free environment. You may not think that eating when you are stressed has any effect on your weight, but you're wrong. It can have a hugely detrimental effect.

If you eat when you're stressed it can lead to something called 'hurried woman syndrome'. This is a throwback to the fight-or-flight situation where (back in the days when we were chased around by bears) we were faced with stressful situation and had to either fight or flee. When we are stressed, our bodies produce adrenaline to prepare us for action ahead (in the past, this would be fighting or fleeing). All of our body's energies are directed to the brain and muscles, which will be required to

169

cope with the perceived danger. This means that other parts of the body do not get the oxygen and glucose they need, thereby suppressing processes that are considered to be 'non-emergency'. Digestion is not a priority in a stressful situation, so it effectively closes down, and works far less efficiently. In the past, of course, our ancestors would have fought or fled, and dispersed the adrenaline building up in their bodies. Their systems would soon return to normal, and digestion and other important processes would restart.

Today, the stress we face is rather different (such as missing a train or the last pair of Louboutin stilettos in the sale), and our bodies have to deal with all of the adrenaline that is floating around our bodies. We tend not to do something physical to disperse it, so it is eventually stored and turned into fat that sits around our midriff. Every woman's worst nightmare!

The term 'hurried woman syndrome' was first coined by the US gynaecologist Dr Brent Bost, who applied it to women (who tend to be between 25 and 55) who are trying to do too much. Weight gain is only one of the symptoms. Others include tiredness, increased appetite, insomnia, low sex drive, lack of motivation, and feelings of guilt and low self-esteem. So, it's truly something to avoid. Bost has written a whole book about the syndrome, and provided seven helpful steps to a hurried-woman-syndrome-free you. But what we are concerned with here is avoiding stress because of its impact on the digestive system. So as well as chewing properly, eating well early at breakfast time, having a light and early dinner, and avoiding raw food after four, it is crucial that all of these are undertaken in a stress-free atmosphere.

Stress-free eating

Try to make time to eat all your meals in calm and peace. Really think about the fact that you are about to nourish your body and it is not a task to be taken lightly. Similarly, avoid eating while arguing, watching the latest terrorist attacks on television, or running from the train to your office.

'Show some respect to the ritual of eating,' says Dr Stossier, 'some respect to nature that has provided us with the food, to the people who have produced the food, and finally some respect to ourselves by eating it in the best way possible. Just make the decision to do this and then it's very easy to follow.'

Try to adopt a French attitude to eating, which involves making it a priority. You would never catch a Frenchman (or woman for that matter) wolfing down a sandwich at the computer. The French make a conscious effort to sit down and eat a proper meal; for them it means more than just making sure your body is fed. It is an event. When we first moved to France, I remember that an electrician who came to our home to sort out some wiring was horrified to see we didn't eat with the children (then aged one and two). For the French, eating together as a family is crucial. For me, eating with a one- and a two-year old who are busy stuffing peas up their noses was way too stressful.

You need to create an environment that is right for you when it comes to eating. That is all well and good, I hear you protest, but if you're trying to get three children ready for school, make their packed lunches, help with the homework they forgot to do the night before, remember the gym kit, get dressed yourself and find the car keys, that doesn't really leave much time for a tranquil and zen breakfast, does it? This is unfortunate, as breakfast should be the day's most important meal. What does Dr Stossier suggest?

'Of course I understand that it is difficult, but it is a question of deciding what your priorities are,' he says. 'Getting up half an hour earlier so you can start the day as you mean to go on, in terms of nourishing your body and ensuring your long-term health, isn't much of a sacrifice, is it?'

I suppose he has a point. But what happens if there really is no other option? If it's a question of wolfing something down or not eating at all?

'Don't eat at all,' says Dr Stossier. 'We all eat far too much anyway.

'Eating in a hurry means we don't chew well, we don't produce enough saliva, and fermentation and putrification occur in our guts. It's just not worth it.'

If you're stressed, don't eat

Nowadays I often have to eat lunch after three. My children finish school at 1.40, and I need to be there to collect them. That means leaving the office at one. If I have lunch before I leave, I have found I end up in a mad rush to leave on time. So I have decided to have a mid-morning snack of some almonds or fruit (or both), and to eat lunch when I'm back in the office, and don't need to be thinking about rushing off anywhere.

Rushing is, in fact, a form of stress, and Dr S recommends, simply, that we avoid eating in that situation. If your body is under stress, it is busy coping with that stress, and will not be in a position to digest properly. It is no accident that when we are stressed, we lose our appetite. Whoever heard of anyone who has just been in a car crash wanting anything more than a strong cup of tea?

Stress is not only psychological, either. There are other

stressors that we simply can't control, such as air pollution, toxins in our food, physical pain, hormonal swings and even noise. All these things will deter optimum digestion. Tiredness is also another form of stress; therefore, if you have a long working day, you will not only be physically tired, but your digestive function will be weaker as well.

We need to support our bodies by keeping stress under control, and this means reducing exposure to things that are stressful, and also learning some coping strategies. When Dr Stossier examined me and my pot belly, he announced that I was severely exhausted and stressed, and that's why he prescribed my 'one hour a day, one day a week, and one month a year' regeneration time. According to Dr Stossier, we maintain our health by recharging our batteries through activity or even inactivity. And it is amazing how much better I feel if I do get that hour a day, either reading a book, having a manicure, or going to the gym.

Stress and mood

My mood has always been closely linked to my digestion. My digestive system has been below par for as long as I can remember. For example, as a child it would block up as soon as I got nervous. When I am stressed, I immediately experience stomach cramps. To me, this proves the close connection between mood and digestion. If I get a nasty letter from the bank, I can feel my stomach bloating almost as I read the words 'unauthorised overdraft'. The result is that I am bloated and crabby as hell. I seem to have passed this malaise on to my middle daughter. I am constantly feeding her prunes in an effort to give her digestion a helping hand – and hopefully improve her behaviour!

My grandmother used to say that as long as your insides

are working well, everything else is, too. The Arabs call the intestine the 'father of mood swings'. And there is also a Latin phrase stating that we can't 'study' on a full stomach.

Dr Stossier believes that in the same way that our physical health is inextricably linked to our digestion, our mental health is, too.

'We could empty all the psychiatric departments of the world, if we would just treat the bellies of these patients,' says Dr Stossier, citing a Nobel prize-winner and Viennese psychiatrist Julius Wagner Jauregg. 'In modern medicine, we are at last beginning to acknowledge the huge link between the belly and the mind.'

For example, about 30 per cent of us suffer from a condition known as 'fructose malabsorption', caused by an inflammation of the intestines, which means that our enzymes are unable to digest and absorb sugar from fruit (known as fructose). As a consequence, our intake of the amino acid tryptophan is reduced, and we produce less of the hormone serotonin, which is known as the 'happy hormone'. Anyone suffering from fructose malabsorption will experience mood swings. Very often, says Dr Stossier, his clients report that they have been eating healthily and feel worse for it. Could this be you? Try eating some fruit and see how you feel afterwards. Do you feel bloated? Depressed? If so, you could be suffering from this condition, and it's something that even the most powerful antidepressants won't touch. The simple solution is to stop eating fruit, after which your symptoms will disappear.

This kind of maldigestion is very often related to a parasite problem such as worms, lambliasis (caused by the parasite Giardia lamblia), or even candida, like my friend Annie at the clinic has, which has to be treated by avoiding certain foods. After three months on a strict diet, you should be able to resume eating fruit, as your body builds up enough enzymes to digest fruit sugar properly again.

The fertility link

Fertility is another area that is hugely affected by stress. According to Dr Stossier (and there are many Viva Mayr babies, who are evidence that his theories are correct), infertility is linked to stress.

'If you are stressed, you cannot reproduce,' he says. 'You have no desire for sex or reproduction, which obviously impacts on your ability to become pregnant in the first place. Think about it in terms of animals in the wild; they will hardly be copulating when they're trying to stay alive.'

In stressful situations, our bodies think we have to fight or flee to stay alive, and in neither situation is copulation or subsequent impregnation likely or ideal. As a consequence of stress, our adrenal glands produce more cortisone, while levels of sex hormones are decreased. The reason for this is that most oestrogens, as well as progesterone and testosterone, are all produced in our adrenal glands, alongside adrenaline and cortisone. When we are in a stressful situation, the production of adrenaline and cortisone takes priority.

According to Dr Stossier, if you are having trouble getting pregnant, the first thing to do is to locate where the stress is coming from and deal with it. The reason is that if your adrenals are working on producing adrenaline and cortisone to cope with stress, your body won't be able to produce the optimal amount and balance of hormones necessary to conceive.

Another possible reason for infertility could be a chronic inflammatory condition caused by fermentation and a toxic overload in the gut (see page 103). The uterus and the lower intestine share a space in the lower abdomen, so if the lower intestine is inflamed, we run the risk that the inflammation will extend into the uterus and the ovaries. As a result, the body will try to distance the uterus from the sick intestine, in order to protect it. In this situation, we unwittingly move our hips backwards. It might look sexy, but it's not healthy.

The inflammation may also irritate the tissue of the uterus, which will hinder conception. Why? Because it is difficult for an inseminated egg to find a good place to develop in tissue that is inflamed.

Higher cholesterol levels

We have all been encouraged to avoid high cholesterol levels, as high levels have been linked with serious heart disease (leading to a heart attack) and stroke. While it is important to avoid high-cholesterol foods, it is equally important to consider our stress levels, which Dr Stossier claims can also raise cholesterol levels.

I once had a boyfriend who suffered from high cholesterol. Halfway through dinner with him, I would often lose the will to live. He checked every single little detail of everything single thing he ate; he ordered food with no fat at all, fiddled about for ages, and then finally ate almost nothing. It drove me mad. Apparently, just like me with my sit-ups, all this was a total waste of time as well.

'Cholesterol is related much more to stress than to food. I can guarantee that for a person with high cholesterol, around 50 per cent of the problem is going to be due to stress,' says Dr Stossier. 'One way the body regulates stress is to produce more cholesterol, so that we have enough to produce the cortisone we need. So you can forget about eating all the right things; what you need to do is reduce your stress levels.'

Dr Stossier is backed up by a recent experiment in Austria, where doctors studied two groups of patients – one with high cholesterol and another without. Each group was asked about stress levels. The group with high cholesterol said they had experienced a lot of stress, while the low-cholesterol group recorded less stress. They then spend four weeks on a typical Austrian cure at a spa or clinic enjoying various treatments. The only difference was that they were allowed to eat and drink anything they wanted to. Unbeknown to the patients, the researchers arranged to expose them to a variety of foods with a higher level of cholesterol than nutritionists recommend.

At the end of four weeks, the high-cholesterol group had benefited hugely and their cholesterol levels were way down, despite the fact that they had been eating everything they wanted – including foods with high cholesterol levels.

'They were relaxed, they had reduced their stress levels due to the healing experience, and they were having fun. They were also not worrying about what they ate,' says Dr Stossier. He does concede that making dietary adjustments is important, such as increasing your intake of unsaturated fatty acids in the form of omega oils (omega 3, in particular; see pages 43–5), and ensuring that you get good levels of fibre, zinc, magnesium, and vitamins A, B3 and B5 in your diet. However, first and foremost, you should deal with your stress levels, as this will have the most dramatic and profound effect.

Eating for health

The ancient Greeks believed that we have two choices relating to our eating habits. We can eat to stay healthy, or eat to become ill. This may seem obvious, but what you may not have considered is the fact that *how* we eat is as important as *what* we eat, in relation to our health and well-being. If we eat the right thing in the right way, we are helping our to bodies stay healthy; if we don't, we do the opposite.

For me, it's a simple equation. If I eat properly and at the right times, my pot belly vanishes. If I don't, I end up bloated, uncomfortable and miserable. Even worse (although there are few things that are worse than a pot belly), I could end up with a chronic illness, such as a heart attack, diabetes or cancer. Although you may not have the pot belly issues that I endured all my life until I met Dr Stossier, you must also make the decision to eat well for a healthy and thin future – whatever your particular nemesis.

How stress affects weight

For as long as we can remember, human beings have suffered from stress. Today, we define stress as being the culmination (or summary) of all of the things that influence us, from inside our bodies and out. Stress also involves our physiological reaction to these stressors. Therefore, stress (in other words, stressors) is not the only problem, but it includes our reaction to it, too.

The aim of the stress reaction (see above) was to survive and stay alive. The adrenaline and cortisone that was pumped out gave us the physical ability to do that, and shutting down or sidelining non-essential body functions meant that our brains and muscles were geared up for action. The stress reaction is managed by our adrenal glands, small organs above our kidneys where we produce both cortisone and adrenaline. These hormones are responsible for ensuring that our metabolism has the energy we need to survive. Energy is, effectively, sugar, and so one of their primary roles is to increase the sugar levels in our blood, which we will need in a fight-or-flight situation.

So, you can imagine that if we are stressed more or less all of the time, we will not only have increased levels of these two hormones, but we will also have an increased level of blood sugar, known as glucose. In this case, another hormone swings into action. This is insulin, which is produced in the pancreas to regulate our blood sugar levels. We have already discovered the function of insulin in the body (see page 41); in a nutshell, when we have enough insulin in our body, it encourages us to store any excess as fat. So in cases of permanent stress, when blood glucose levels are high, we have loads of insulin being produced. And because of this insulin, our bodies are unable to use the fat from our stores; instead, the insulin levels must be reduced *first*. In order to do this, we must not only reduce our stress levels (or at least manage them), but we also need to reduce our intake of carbohydrates, which provide *more* sugar that is subsequently laid down as fat.

In the Stone Age, faster and stronger men and women survived. They confronted stress and after the stressful situation had passed, they took time to regenerate. Our adrenal glands are not designed to produce consistently high levels of hormones; we could never be in fight or flight mode all the time. We would become exhausted, and our adrenal glands would be unable to respond properly to real threats. In this situation, we experience overwhelming exhaustion and inertia, known as 'burn-out'. For that reason, at Viva Mayr it is suggested that time is *always* taken to regenerate and to ensure that our adrenal glands are working at optimum level. To do this, they need a rest. And when they get that rest, weight problems can be avoided and weight loss can occur.

Top tips for reducing stress in your life

Try to stay positive. For example, if you are stuck in a traffic jam and running late, choose to stay calm. Think: *There is nothing I can do about this, so I am not going to worry. I'm going to use this lovely, peaceful time to think about anything I want.* Or put on Robert Palmer's 'Addicted to Love', and crank up the volume. You can't stay stressed for long when you are singing along to *that*!

Breathe. This is crucially important. If you feel yourself getting stressed, do some yoga breathing – in and out through your nose. Breathe in for the count of four, and then out for the count of six.

I have spent most of my life worrying about things that never happened. Try to avoid this. If you've got something on your mind, ask yourself, rationally, if it is real or the result of an overactive imagination. Worrying is a waste of time, and very stressful.

Remember to choose calm – you can let things get to you, go AWOL, and raise your blood pressure and stress levels, or you can go zen and cope. It may sound simplistic, but we are empowered by the right and the ability to make choices.

Try to laugh! It's one of the best things you can do, improving circulation, boosting immunity, and acting as an anti-ageing agent. Better still, it helps to disperse the build-up of adrenaline in the body.

Get active. In the Stone Age, the physical act of fighting or fleeing caused the adrenaline floating around our bodies to be discharged. Today, we sit at our desks or on the sofa, stressing away with no outlet. Exercise gets rid of the adrenaline, so get out there and run it off. It will lift your mood, too!

In summary ...

Stress is one of the single most detrimental influences on our health, and it affects everything from our moods and fertility to our weight and cholesterol levels.

It's better to eat nothing at all than to eat in stressful circumstances.

Learning to cope with stress rather than simply trying to reduce the number of stressful situations is the best approach.

Case Study

Samantha, 42, London

I was very different from most of the people who go to Viva Mayr, in that I went there to be completely replenished, instead of trying to get rid of excess weight or some illness. I was in my late 30s and had spent 15 years not taking very good care of myself. I was constantly travelling, on the road for ten months of the year, and not getting much sleep. I am a journalist and was working for aid agencies in war zones, where I just had to eat what was available. So even though I knew how to eat healthily, there were times when I couldn't.

My system was really run down. Because my adrenal glands were working so fiercely when I was working due to the stress, I wouldn't get sick at the time but when I came back I would literally collapse. I would pick up whatever anyone around me had – every kind of infection going. Even if a mosquito bit me, I'd get an infection. I constantly had bronchitis. I was really a wreck. I went to see a doctor in London who told me that I had dangerously compromised my immune system because I was so broken down and overworked.

By the time I decided I wanted to have a baby, it was pretty clear that my body was no place to host a pregnancy. I managed to get pregnant fairly easily, but I suffered from recurrent miscarriages at around ten or twelve weeks. In one year,

I suffered three. So, in addition to having a stressed out body, I also had a pretty nasty hormonal imbalance.

One of my best friends is Austrian and she told me about Viva Mayr. It is just part of her life, and she goes there every year. She suggested that it would be the ideal place for me to unwind and regenerate. And so I went there after a five-month stint in Iraq. I was getting married and really wanted to get pregnant again. Dr Stossier said I should stay for two weeks.

The first week was really tough. I felt terrible and I got very depressed — so much so, that I even wanted to leave, I felt lost without work every day — I missed my phone ringing — and struggled to let go. But, by the second week, I was totally into the rhythm of it and the thought of the real world was terrifying. I ended up staying for a total of five weeks.

Dr Stossier and his team really replenished everything that had been wiped out. I was on the Viva Mayr Diet but I was also given vitamins and minerals through an intravenous drip. By the end of it, I felt as if I had been taken and scrubbed from the inside out — as if I had been given a transfusion of new blood or something.

When it was time to leave, Dr Stossier said: 'This time you will get pregnant and it will stay.' He said it with complete confidence. I had never heard that from a doctor before.

I got back to London and went to a party, feeling so disconnected. Stuffing myself with foods that I knew weren't good for me seemed so alien. But, about a month later, I got pregnant and it stuck. That was my miracle baby. My Mayr baby.

All the reading that I did while I was at the clinic showed me that my adrenal system is extremely closely linked to my reproductive system, and that something was blocked. I just didn't have the energy to sustain a pregnancy before I went there. I really feel Viva Mayr changed my life, not just because of my lovely baby boy, but I firmly believe that their treatment has halted the terrible genetic pattern of cancer in our family that my siblings and my father died from. I go back to Viva Mayr every year now to top up on the way of life.

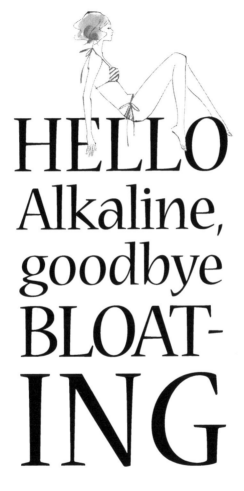

HELLO
Alkaline,
goodbye
BLOAT-
ING

You are about to discover:

The importance of maintaining a healthy acid–alkaline balance

How to combine your food to achieve that balance

How to say goodbye to bloating – forever

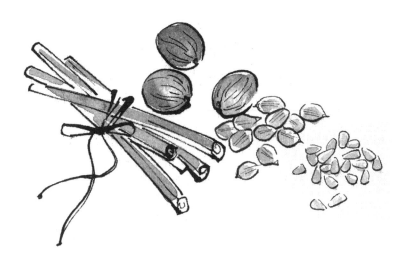

Today's Menu

Breakfast:
Green tea, and papaya and banana salad with cinnamon yoghurt and almond purée (see page 265)

Lunch
Potato roulade with beetroot, broccoli and parsley oil, and banana mousse (see pages 266–7)

Dinner
Cream of artichoke base soup with Mediterranean vegetable spread and spelt bread (see page 268)

I remember the evening my husband and I decided to try for a third child. We were in a beach restaurant in Montpellier.

'Shall we have another baby?' I asked.

My husband looked at me. To be honest, I was expecting a 'no, don't be so bloody ridiculous'. We already had two girls, added to which my husband had a girl and a boy from his previous marriage. Four children is a lot by anyone's standards.

He took a sip of his wine. 'As long as it's a boy,' he said.

'OK,' I replied immediately, although I had absolutely no idea what I was going to do to determine the sex of our baby. I just thought quietly to myself that it must be possible. And if it turned out to be a girl – well, it would all be too late by then anyway. And at least we already had lots of girls' clothes.

The next day I started to find out what I could do to ensure that my husband didn't regret his decision – or 'moment of madness', as he called it that morning when he woke up with a bit of a hangover. Not surprisingly, I discovered that the sex of your child, like just about everything else, can be influenced by what you eat.

According to www.genderlabs.com, a not-for-profit website, which promises that you can 'pre-select the gender of your baby naturally', the first thing to do is to change your eating habits. For a boy, you need an alkaline environment; for a girl, it should be acid. So the diet for a boy is based on foods like potatoes, which are high in sodium and potassium. The diet for a girl is based on dairy products and meat; both proteins that are high in acid.

It all comes down to the acid–alkaline balance in your stomach, and this is something that forms a big part of the Viva Mayr Diet. One of the goals of the Viva Mayr Diet is to balance acid and alkaline (or 'base', as Dr S calls it) foods in our diet. This means reducing animal protein (meat, fish and cheese) in favour of vegetables, potatoes and cold-pressed vegetable oils. These recommendations for restoring an acid-base balance go hand in hand with the Viva Mayr suggestion that we should reduce our intake of meat and fish to a maximum of every other day. Not only will this reduce your intake of acidic foods, but it will mean you have more room for alkaline or 'base' foods.

And this is the focus of Day Twelve. You need to redress your acid–alkaline balance and learn how to create the best possible environment in your gut for health, longevity and, of course, becoming and staying slim.

A word about acid …

Did you know that almost all poisons are, more or less, acids? Furthermore, most chronic diseases are related to acid in some way. And when there is too much acid, the result is pain. For example, gout is caused by uric acid; pain in our muscles following a heavy workout is caused by a build-up of lactic acid. So, it looks as though acid isn't a good thing.

However, we *do* need acid to digest our food. In fact, as soon as we start thinking about eating, acids start forming to deal with the food we are about to swallow. So how do we strike a balance that is good for digestion, without causing any health problems?

Acids are extremely aggressive, and will attack and destroy body tissue, given half a chance. Our stomach is the only organ that can produce large amounts of acid and, fortunately, it is protected by something known as 'epithelial cells', which produce and secrete a bicarbonate-rich solution that coats the mucous membrane lining. So while the stomach is busy producing hydrochloric acid (which digests our food), from water, carbon dioxide and salt, it also produces the 'antidote' to this – which is required to prevent the stomach from actually digesting itself! So even in the most acidic organ in the body, both acid and alkaline must be in balance in order for the stomach to function.

The essential acid–alkaline balance

This balance is a major regulator, not only in the human body, but throughout nature. Pollution, acid rain and chemicals in the environment affect our global acid–alkaline balance, rotting the planet, in much the same way that too much acidic food rots our insides. For example, damage to forests is, in part, caused by overly acidic soils, which have been affected by environmental factors; and, as every farmer knows, you can't get high yields from a field with 'sour' or acidic soil. Obviously the focus of this section is to establish the importance of the acid–alkaline balance in our bodies; however, you can see how an imbalance can affect the world around us as well.

Believe it or not, there is a book called *Alkalize or Die*, by Theodore A. Baroody, an American doctor. His theory is that 'the countless names of illnesses do not really matter. What does matter is that they all come from the same root cause ... too much tissue acid waste in the body!'

In fact, the list of illnesses linked to a poor acid–alkaline balance (otherwise known as the pH balance), or 'acidosis', makes for depressing reading. Acidity is linked to all of the following conditions:

- Cardiovascular diseases.

- Weight gain, obesity and diabetes.

- Bladder and kidney disorders, including kidney stones.

- Poor immunity.

- Free-radical damage (see pages 207–8), which can potentially lead to some cancers.

- Hormone problems.

- Premature ageing (*eeek*).

- Osteoporosis (weakening of the bones, which become brittle and subject to fractures).

- Joint pain, aching muscles and lactic acid build-up (see page 195).

- Low energy and chronic fatigue.

- Slow digestion and elimination.

- Yeast/fungal overgrowth (like candida, which poor Annie had).

Acid in our diet

Protein is one of the most acidic foods – especially animal protein, such as meat, fish and cheese. Meat and fish contain about 20 per cent pure protein, and cheese can have as much as 35 per cent. Legumes (or 'pulses' – for example, peas, beans, lentils and soya) also contain 30 per cent or more pure protein, which puts even vegetarians who eat large amounts of these foods at risk of taking in too much acid.

Food-processing is also a key factor in making food acid. Industrially processed, tinned or preserved foods tend to be more acidic than the foods from which they are made. So, for example, fresh peas would be far less acidic than tinned peas in sugar and salt.

Fats also require special attention in this context. Oils are extremely important to a healthy diet, and should be eaten in virtually unlimited quantities; however, when they are industrially produced they become acidic, which means they simply shouldn't be eaten. That's one reason why choosing cold-pressed, organic oils is so important.

You may also be disappointed to learn that alcoholic beverages and coffee belong on the list of acid foods…

Alkaline foods

Alkaline-producing foods include all vegetables, as well as cold-pressed, virgin nut, seed and vegetable oils. Vegetables – and, in particular, potatoes – have a low protein content (usually between 1 and 3 per cent), which enables their alkaline (or 'base') content to predominate.

Many fruits are alkaline-producing, provided they are properly ripened. Fruits store many vital nutrients during the ripening process, which normally takes place outdoors, and in the natural sunlight. However, if fruit is ripened artificially, or harvested unripe, it's unlikely to contain these important nutrients, and will have a more acidic effect in the body.

Milk and cream are alkaline-producing foods, which may seem odd, given that other dairy produce, such as cheese, is acid-producing. Cream and milk contain only about 3 per cent protein, and they are very rich in unsaturated fatty acids, as well as key minerals, such as calcium. However, when we produce cheese from milk, we concentrate the protein, thereby creating an acid food.

Herbs and spices are also alkaline (base) foods. Even though their alkaline content is not very significant, and they are used only in small quantities, they are nevertheless important for healthy nutrition. They contain essential oils, bitter substances that promote digestive capacity, as well as specific plant compounds that impart healthy benefits.

Acid and alkaline (base) foods

Acidic

Meat and fish

Dairy products, cheese

Grains

Pulses (beans, peas, etc.)

Citrus fruit

Refined and processed foods

Animal fats

Refined oils

Alcoholic beverages

Coffee and tea

Alkaline (base)

Vegetables

Potatoes

Cold-pressed vegetable oils

Local, ripe fruit

Milk, cream

Herbs, spices

Nuts, seeds

If you eat the Viva Mayr way, your acid-base balance should be in good shape. Unhealthy eating habits – such as eating more food than our digestive systems can handle at any one time – cause impaired digestion, which adversely affects our acid-base balance. But you also need to be aware of how to combine your food so you don't create more acid than your body needs. In excess, acid can be damaging.

For example, eating a lot of raw vegetables, such as salads, or fruit, can lead to increased acid levels because of the fermentation process to which they are prone (see page 103). At the same time, these foods are our most important alkaline contributors. So we need to make sure we eat them at the right time of day (before four), otherwise they can turn acid (when not digested properly). This is technically known as 'the reverse impact of base foods'; something we need to avoid, even if we don't necessarily need to remember the term itself!

Combining foods

As well as eating the right thing at the right time, we need to avoid combining foods that will create an acid environment. The goal of a healthy diet and acid–alkaline balance is not to avoid acidic foods entirely. This would not only be impossible but it would also be unwise, because we do need some acid in our diets for digestion and other body processes. The important thing is getting the balance right. And that's what the Viva Mayr Diet does very well.

As a rule, our bodies maintain a slightly alkaline environment, especially inside our cells. Blood is also alkaline and only a few organs, such as our stomach, are able to tolerate acid without incurring damage. When you choose what to eat, and how to combine your food, try to achieve a two to one alkaline to acid ratio. In other words, eat two alkaline foods for every one acid food you eat. You also need to avoid eating combinations of several acidic foods in any one meal. See the tables below for clarification of this concept.

Undesirable food combinations

Meat, fish +   Rice, noodles, pasta, grains, cheese, eggs

Ideal combinations

Meat, fish		Salads
Grains	**+**	Vegetables, vegetable soups
Noodle/pasta dishes		and sauces
		Potatoes
		Herbs
		Ripe fruit
		Cold-pressed vegetable oils

What about portions?

While there are no hard and fast rules about portion sizes on the Viva Mayr Diet, it is important to keep on eye on how much acidic food you eat. The reason is that acidic foods are normally more concentrated – rather like using a concentrated washing liquid rather than your usual brand. This means you need two portions of alkaline foods, such as potatoes and cooked vegetables, to balance the effects of one acid one, such as a steak.

Ideally, you should try to maintain this 2:1 proportion at every meal, but don't panic if you don't. We usually have enough alkaline reserves to keep the balance. But overdoing it on the acid front, particularly long term, will lead to health problems, and that's precisely what we want to avoid.

Have a few 'balancing days', like today, when you eat primarily alkaline or vegetarian foods to regenerate your 'base' reserves. When you are preparing meals, look at the tables above and choose a breakfast, lunch and dinner that is purely alkaline, such as pasta with steamed broccoli, or baked potatoes with ratatouille. Chose from vegetables high in alkaline content, like broccoli, spinach, root vegetables and asparagus, to make a soup, or go for a salad, and sprinkle some high-alkaline almonds on top. Other days, try to go for double the number of alkaline foods in relation to the acid foods you eat. It's easy, I promise; and there is plenty to choose from in both categories.

Goodbye bloating

So what about that awful bloated feeling? Sometimes I have it, and it is so nasty that my stomach swells up as tight as a drum and I feel (and look) about nine months' pregnant. Is it the ghastly

IBS or Irritable Bowel Syndrome, I ask Dr S? IBS is something I have long been convinced I have, but am always unsure of what it is. Apparently around eight million people in the UK have it.

'Bloating and IBS are both basically an acid situation,' explains Dr Stossier. 'What happens is that excess stomach acid attacks the stomach's mucous membranes, which can cause gastritis [irritation of the lining], as well as stomach ulcers. The stomach protects itself from attacks by stomach acid by producing mucus. This mucus is produced by specialised cells [see above] and completely coats the inside of our stomach. If the balance between mucus and acid is disturbed, and excess acid is present, the acid damages the mucous membranes, causing inflammation and pain.'

When that happens, we can try to reduce the acidity by eating different – and preferably alkaline – foods. The excess acid will be neutralised to some extent. However, when we neutralise the acid, carbon dioxide is produced, which is a gas, and can cause bloating. In many cases, a bloated belly is caused by an imbalance in the small or large intestine, where fermenting (of too many carbs, for example) creates gas and, you guessed it, bloating.

So all we need to do is avoid acid?

'Well, up to a point,' says Dr S. 'If there is not enough stomach acid present, protein digestion is not properly initiated. This can cause digestive problems and allergies, especially if medications to block acid are used.'

Given the importance of acid–alkaline balance for our health, we should be aware about other sources of acidity. Our diet is obviously the most important source, but it is by no means the only factor affecting our acid–alkaline balance. Intense physical work or exercise, for example, creates large amounts of acids. When we over-exert ourselves, our muscles can't get enough oxygen to meet the high energy requirements and this creates lactic acid, which accumulates in our muscles, causing them to ache. If we constantly over-exert ourselves and cause acidosis, we risk muscle injury. This often occurs in sportsmen and sportswomen, where over-exertion can lead to torn muscles or even injured ligaments. Obviously I am not suggesting you don't exercise, but try not to overdo it every day. Have a rest day in between, to give the acid a chance to dissipate.

Other ways to establish a balance

In fact, exercise is very good for our acid–alkaline balance. When you exercise, you breathe more heavily. In every breath we eliminate carbon dioxide from our bodies, which is an acid. So it makes sense that exercise encourages and enhances this process. In fact, exhaling acid is the best and most effective way to eliminate acids. Since I learned this, I have managed to get rid of some bloating simply by breathing deeply.

Relaxing is another important way to maintain your acid–alkaline balance. Generally speaking, any type of stress can lead to acidosis, whether it is emotional or physical. So making an effort to reduce stressors and to cope better with stress (see page 180) can make a dramatic different.

Furthermore, a number of classic metabolic disorders also lead to increased acidosis; these include diabetes, inflammatory diseases such as arthritis, auto-immune conditions, gum inflammation and chronic bowel inflammation. So how do you know if you have it? Acidosis shows up in many different areas of the body with a variety of very different symptoms. This is because the various tissues in our body each have different functions. The major signs to look out for include:

- A coating on your tongue, which can be either milky-white or yellow-brown to dark brown. Not a good look.

- A spotty tongue, which indicates that your liver has been trying to eliminate acids and toxins for some time.

- Tooth impressions on the sides of your tongue, which is a sign of an acid–alkaline imbalance and an inflammation of the small intestine, as well as lymphatic disorders.

- Deep cracks in the tongue, which is always a sign of chronic acidosis.

Becoming more alkaline

Inside out …

Our bodies cannot produce alkaline on their own, so we need to ingest it. The very simplest and cheapest way to do this is to use sodium bicarbonate (also known as baking soda), which neutralises acids – much in the same way that the bicarb in the lining of our stomachs does. Dissolve one level teaspoon of bicarbonate of soda in 250ml of warm water, to create a milky solution. If it tastes too strong, use a little less bicarb but the same amount of water. Drink this solution between meals *only*. During meals, we need concentrated digestive juices and an acidic environment for our stomachs to digest properly. The last thing you need to do at this point is dilute the acids!

Drinking this solution in the evening before bedtime is especially beneficial because it supports the work of our liver. Our liver performs its peak detoxification work during the night, and to do so, it requires a large amount of alkaline substances (or base). This can be supplied by drinking the bicarbonate of soda mixture, or a 'base powder solution', which is a little more powerful as it contains added minerals to reduce cell acidity. This can be purchased directly from Viva Mayr; see page 282).

If you suffer from recurrent symptoms of acidosis, you can drink the bicarbonate of soda mixture, or a base powder solution, several times a day. It may cause some burping, so beware! The minerals in the base powder solution from Viva Mayr, including potassium and magnesium, can help to relieve cramps and reduce muscle tension, as well as help to ease constipation, heart problems, high blood pressure and more.

... and outside in

A good way to remove acids via the skin is to take a 'base bath', which can easily be done at home. Base (or alkaline) baths support the important elimination work of our skin. Taken regularly (once a week, for example), a base bath will support the acid–alkaline balance, and improve the function of the skin. Once again, the best alkaline substance to use is bicarbonate of soda.

The water temperature should be a comfortable 37°C (98.6°F). Remain in the bath for 30 to 40 minutes for best effect, topping up the tub with warm water to keep the temperature constant. Ideally, you should rest for about an hour after a base bath; for this reason, it's a good idea to take them before bed, so you can simply go to sleep instead of resting.

Scrubbing the body several times with an alkaline soap can help to eliminate acids through the skin. A brush or a massage glove can be used to intensify this application.

You'll be astonished by the 'ring around the tub', which is the visual evidence of how the base bath works. This layer of dirt is the result of the intense elimination of toxins through our skin.

Acid ages you

Acid is extremely ageing. Just like sugar, it affects the connective tissue and the fibres that lend elasticity, vitality and youthful good looks to our skin. Acid is temporarily stored in our connective tissue, which leads to decreased elasticity and skin tone and eventually to wrinkles.

It goes without saying that we all have to age; however, if our metabolism is overly acidic, the ageing process is accelerated and intensified. Our nails and hair, which are closely connected with our skin, also become less elastic, our hair loses its sheen, and our nails become brittle or develop spots. What's more, acidosis can lead to uncomfortable swelling, fluid deposits in the joints and muscle tension. Initially, these may be treated with massage or heat application, but the worse it gets, the more permanent they become, because our bodies lose their ability to compensate.

Step by step, acidosis extends to larger areas of the body, causing muscles to shorten and stiffen, and impacting overall mobility. Our initial response to such symptoms may be 'Now I am getting old'. A more appropriate response would be 'Now I am turning sour (acidic)', because it is possible to age without suffering from acidosis, and to maintain one's vitality and mobility well into advanced age.

Prolonged acidosis eventually leads to long-term depletion of calcium and other minerals from our bones. This demineralisation process causes osteoporosis, another typical degenerative disease. Preventing osteoporosis requires not only calcium supplementation, but also the restoration of the acid–alkaline balance through eating the right way. Because cheese is an acidic food, it can't restore the balance our bodies need even though it is rich in calcium, but choosing milk and cream is a good option, as well as leafy green vegetables, which are both alkaline and calcium rich.

The best way to beat osteoporosis

A great study undertaken at the University of Zürich in Switzerland showed the effect of alkaline and acid food intake on the metabolism of calcium, which is required for strong, healthy bones (and teeth). Two groups were compared. One group ate more or less traditional food, with plenty of animal protein such as meat, fish and cheese. The second group ate a vegetarian diet. The researchers then measured how much calcium was eliminated in the urine of both groups.

Amazingly, after four days, the amount of calcium in the traditional-food group was 70 per cent higher than in the vegetarian group. What does that mean? Basically, that protein intake has a dramatic effect upon our acid–alkaline balance, and that it affects how much calcium actually reaches our bones (instead of being peed out!). Interestingly, too, it shows that cheese – which many people eat to prevent osteoporosis because of its high calcium content – had the opposite effect.

In fact, if you simply restore your acid – alkaline balance, you can *stop* the development of osteoporosis. And the same applies to other disorders caused by acidosis, such as heart and circulatory disorders, auto-immune conditions, metabolic problems such as diabetes, and local acid disorders of the stomach, such as gastritis and ulcers.

Even more interesting is the fact that acidosis often causes non-specific, general symptoms such as decreased energy, fatigue, exhaustion and loss of concentration. With all of these conditions, targeted alkaline therapy can restore balance. Sounds good to me! Anything that can help to halt the degenerative effects of ageing can only be a good thing, and that's what we're going to look at in more detail now.

And, in case you're wondering, I did have a boy.

In summary ...

We should aim to eat more alkaline than acid foods – at a ratio of 2:1, if possible.

Having a totally 'alkaline day', once a month, can help to address any excess acidity and re-establish the balance.

Stress can cause acid creation in our bodies, as can over-exertion.

Regular exercise will, however, reduce acidity, as we breathe out the acid gas carbon dioxide when we exhale.

Drinking several litres a day of water, herbal teas or vegetable broth (which are non-acidic liquids) will help to maintain the balance.

Cut down your portion sizes of acidic foods.

Use base powder to restore balance.

Case Study

Jenny, 34, Bristol

By my early thirties, I was overweight and had got to the stage where I could hardly look at food without becoming bloated. As if being too fat wasn't bad enough, I now had a great big gas-filled tummy to deal with as well. I tried several diets but none worked. Then a friend told me about Viva Mayr. I looked into it, read about it, and decided to go to the clinic. I suppose anything was better than the state I was in, but I was amazed at how quick the results were.

It's true that while you are in the clinic, you aren't really doing anything other than focusing on your digestion and relaxing, but still I was impressed. The base powder felt as though it was doing me good from the moment I swallowed it. I think it was just what my body needed — a sort of calming, alkaline concoction to wash away the years of acids. I guess I used to eat meat at least once a day. I was brought up with a 'meat and two veg' mother, and I carried on eating that way even when I left home. It wasn't until I got to Austria that I realised I had been over-feeding myself with protein for years.

It's not hard to stop eating too much acid. I just make Mondays, Wednesdays and Fridays my protein days, and then avoid those foods on the other days. Combining proteins is also something I avoid — I've most definitely learned what goes with it ... the hard way. I still get slightly bloated sometimes; in fact, I can almost feel when I have overdone my eating as I swallow the final mouthful. But I have lost two stone in the last six months, and I feel a hundred times better. There is no question of going back to how I was. I have more energy and really feel I am on the right track to long-term weight loss and good health.

LOOKING
and Feeling
YOUN-
GER

You are about to discover:

More about the most powerful antioxidants in food, and how they can slow down the ageing process

How to avoid the enemy of youthful skin: sugar

How to age gracefully, so that you look and feel better than ever

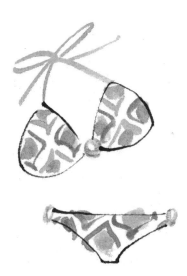

Today's Menu

Breakfast
Malt coffee, and porridge with fresh fruit and linseed oil (see page 269)

Lunch
Mixed leaf salad with yoghurt dressing, and fillet of beef with vegetables and potato cubes (see pages 269–70)

Dinner
Quinoa potato gnocchi with fresh spinach, tomatoes and olive cream (see page 271).

You may have noticed that I have a bit of a weakness for organic shortbread biscuits. In fact, they don't even need to be organic – any shortbread biscuits will do. I am normally quite restrained when it comes to avoiding foods that aren't necessarily good for me, but when faced with a packet of shortbread, well, I just want to eat them all. There is, however, a good reason why I shouldn't, and it is actually sufficiently convincing to prevent me from devouring my favourite treats. I now know that shortbread biscuits, innocent as they may seem, are *ageing*. Yes, you heard me right. These little things are stuffed full of sugar, and if I want young-looking skin, that's about the worst thing I can eat.

There is a whole anti-ageing programme based on eating no sugar, developed by a leading US dermatologist, Dr Frederic Brandt. He says, 'In a nutshell, sugar hastens the degradation of elastin and collagen, both key skin proteins. In other words, it actively ages you.' When he stuck to a sugar-free diet, not only did he lose almost 10 kilos (20-odd pounds), but he saw an increased elasticity and radiance in his face. This was a man who used to drink Orangina every day and eat a tub of ice cream in one sitting!

What's wrong with sugar?

When we eat sugar, it hits the bloodstream and triggers a process called 'glycation', where the sugar molecules bind to our protein fibres (and, in particular, the elastin and collagen fibres in our skin). Imagine that collagen is like the mattress on your bed, and elastin the coils holding it together and giving it 'bounce'. Sugar attacks these fibres, rendering them brittle. Eventually they break. So the 'mattress' of your face has no bounce, and it probably sags, too. The result is most definitely older-looking skin that droops and loses its lustre and 'give'.

As if this isn't bad enough, the glycation process also makes the proteins mutate, and creates damaging molecules called Advanced Glycation End products (AGEs), which also *attack* your collagen and elastin. The result is fine lines and wrinkles. Are they really worth that Mars bar?

Anti-ageing foods

Of course, as well as being ageing, foods can be *anti-ageing*. This is where Viva Mayr comes in. Try to adopt the Viva Mayr habit of thinking about everything you are eating and drinking. Think about whether or not it is actually doing you good. Is it helping you to age better, or making you healthier? If the answer is no, try to avoid it. By Day Thirteen you will already be accustomed to eating healthy, nutrient-packed foods that have a profound effect on your overall health and weight; more to the point, the nutrients they contain will already be hard at work slowing down the degenerative processes of ageing. In fact, making just a few changes to your diet towards the Viva Mayr way can make a dramatic difference to the way you age.

For example, let's say you choose some almonds instead of a Mars bar for dessert. Not only do almonds contain substances that can help to prevent some cancers, including breast, colon and prostate, but they also provide your body with a wealth of vitamins (A, B, C, D and E), minerals (magnesium, phosphorus, zinc and boron), the elusive and magical substance resveratrol (also found in red wine, and linked to reduced incidence of cancer, as well as being a profound antioxidant – the mainstay of healthy ageing), and also folic acid. Not bad for a handful of nuts. Even better, eating almonds five times a week has been found to reduce the risk of heart disease by up to 50 per cent!

Even something as simple as tomato paste (or even tomato ketchup – although watch the sugar) contains an important substance called lycopene, which can help to protect the skin from sun damage. Adapting your diet to ensure that you eat foods that are high in anti-ageing chemicals and antioxidants (see page 208) can make all the difference to your overall health – and looks!

So what are antioxidants?

Antioxidants are substances that may protect your cells against the effects of free radicals. Free radicals are molecules produced when your body breaks down food, or by environmental exposures to substances such as tobacco smoke, toxic chemicals, overexposure to the sun's rays and radiation. Free radicals can damage cells, may play a role in heart disease, cancer and other health conditions, and they are responsible for many of the degenerative effects of ageing, such as less supple skin and arthritic conditions.

Antioxidants are found in all brightly coloured fruits and vegetables (as well as whole grains) and they are often identified in food by their distinctive colours — the deep red of cherries and tomatoes; the orange of carrots; the yellow of corn, mangos, and saffron; and the blue-purple of blueberries, blackberries and grapes. The most well-known components of food with antioxidant activities are vitamins A, C, and E; the minerals selenium and zinc; and more recently, the compound lycopene.

Your anti-ageing, antioxidant shopping list

Almonds (eat them every day), walnuts and any other nuts

Any brightly coloured fruit or vegetables, such as red bell peppers, spinach, sweet potato, aubergines, mangoes, papaya, kiwi fruit and all berries, pomegranates, which are incredibly anti-ageing either in juice, extract or seed form

Avocados

Tomatoes (and anything made from them, such as tomato paste and ketchup)

Stevia (a sugar substitute)

Porridge oats

Sunflower, sesame and pumpkin seeds

Green tea

Organic wild Alaskan sockeye salmon (contains particular nutrients that are extremely good for skin tone and elasticity. There is a famous diet where you eat nothing but this type of fish. Dr Perricone, the founder of said diet, promises you will literally turn back the clock.)

What else can you do?

When you are not eating healthy foods bursting with antioxidants, there are plenty of other things you can do to slow down the process of ageing. The first is to stay out of the sun, or at least wear sun protection every day, even if it's pouring with rain. There are damaging rays in all sorts of light, even artificial light, so protect your face, your décolletage and the backs of your hands at all times. Watch your sunscreen, too. Avoid sunscreens that contain 'nano particles', which are microscopic chemicals (natural and unnatural) that can penetrate our cells and cause damage. All of us do need some sunlight to ensure that our bodies make enough vitamin D to keep our bones healthy and strong, so don't avoid sunlight altogether, and use a sunscreen with a SPF that is appropriate for your colouring.

If you smoke, stop it immediately. Tina Richards, an anti-ageing expert who helped me enormously with my book about ageing, says that smoking is the second most damaging thing to your skin, after the sun. Not only does it rob the body of key nutrients (including antioxidants, and in particular vitamin C, which is required for collagen production), but one study found that cells exposed to smoke produced far more of the enzyme responsible for breaking down skin. Skin stays healthy and young-looking because it has the ability to constantly regenerate itself. This process depends on a subtle balance between the ability to break down old skin and to create fresh replacement tissue. The body breaks down old skin with enzymes called matrix metalloproteinases (MMPs). These enzymes chop up the fibres that form collagen – the tissue that makes up about 80 per cent of normal skin. Research found that cells exposed to smoke produced far more MMP than normal skin cells. This means that skin is broken down far more quickly than it is replaced, causing wrinkles, dry skin, sagging and more!

You also need to exercise a little every day – even if it's just a brisk walk to get your circulation going. Regular exercise can help increase skin tone and maintain elasticity, and it can increase the blood flow to your skin, giving it a healthy glow. Also, body sweat triggers production of sebum, which is the skin's own natural moisturiser.

Exercise reduces stress (see below). One study found that highly stressed people who get little exercise report 21 per cent more anxiety those who exercise more frequently. Exercise works by using up the adrenaline that is created by stress and stressful situations. It also creates 'endorphins', the feel-good hormones that improve mood, motivation and even tolerance to pain and other stimuli. Aerobic exercise helps to increase the number of brain chemicals, called neurotransmitters, so that messages can be carried more quickly over brain cells. This increases mental flexibility and agility over longer periods of time. Furthermore, regular exercise increases the supply of oxygenated blood to the brain, which can improve concentration, alertness and intellectual capacity. We all want sharp brains as we age, so this is one great way to make sure it happens.

Stress is a factor in the ageing process, and that's another reason why it is important to avoid stressors and also to learn how to cope better with them (see page 180). One positive side-effect of reducing our stress load, is better sleep, and this is incredibly important for ageing well. Sleep has a multitude of functions, including overcoming the effects of stress and giving our bodies time to restore and rejuvenate. Furthermore, most cells of the body show increased production and reduced breakdown of proteins during deep sleep, which refreshes the skin and every other cell and organ in the body. On a practical level, you may also want to try sleeping on your back, as sleeping on your side or front creates wrinkles on your face and your décolletage!

Look after your skin

You probably have a good skincare routine already, and it really is an essential part of maintaining healthy, younger-looking skin. One of the things that really ages our skin is dead skin clogging up the pores, so make sure that regular, gentle exfoliation is part of your routine. You should exfoliate your body too, either with an exfoliating cream or body brushing. I use an exfoliating cleanser every morning, but three times a week should be enough. Look out for face creams that actually *contain* anti-oxidants (see pages 207–8) and choose one with active ingredients such as vitamin C or green tea in it.

Growing old gracefully is, in my view, linked to eating. And for me, eating is linked to Viva Mayr. I now make all my culinary decisions with Viva Mayr in mind. For example, I always have a salad for lunch. Not only is this in the Viva Mayr ethos, but it is very anti-ageing, one because I am eating antioxidants and two, because I am eating them at a time when my body can digest them without putting unnecessary strain on my digestive system – which is also anti-ageing.

Growing old gracefully is also about your mental attitude. But as we have seen throughout the book, your state of mind is inexorably linked to your digestive health. So look after that and you will feel great, which in turn equals feeling (and looking) young!

In summary ...

- Eating sugar (particularly in excess) is one of the most damaging things you can do for the health of your skin.

- Ensuring that you get plenty of antioxidant-rich foods on a daily basis will help to slow down the process of ageing.

- Ensuring that you eat and sleep well, get adequate exercise, learn to cope better with stress, and protect your skin will all help you to age well on all levels.

Case Study

Helena (that's me!), 44, Abu Dhabi

When I started to research my book about ageing, I was convinced that the way forward lay in complicated and expensive procedures, like liposuction and Botox. In fact, I tried several of those procedures myself. However, as time went on and I met more and more women who had aged gracefully, I began to realise that the single most important thing affecting the way we age is *what we eat*. You can have as many facelifts as you like, but if you live off Diet Coke and McDonald's you are never going to look good. Eating in an anti-ageing manner is not difficult. It is just as easy as eating things that are bad for you. You can pick up a bag of crisps or a bag of almonds. You can drink a fresh orange juice or a Red Bull. You can eat Coco Pops for breakfast or organic muesli.

There is no mystery to it, and once you understand how vital it is to give your body the right nutrients with which to fight ageing, it becomes very difficult to do anything else. I found that eating for my looks is identical to eating for my health. Tina Richards, an anti-ageing expert and friend once said to me 'Eat to feed your skin'. By this she meant eat things to make your skin glow. And of course these things do not include Krispy Kremes. So by eating to nourish your skin you stay slim and healthy at the same time.

I have made tiny tweaks in the way I eat, for example always choosing something that will be good for me as opposed to something that will not, always saying no to sugar (well, almost always — I do have a piece of dark chocolate every day, but it is 85 per cent cacao) and never drinking caffeine (which is dehydrating and therefore ageing, because a lot of the signs of ageing are caused by loss of moisture). But I promise I have not become a bore and I don't find eating like this boring either. It has now just become habit and as with most habits, good or bad, it's hard to break. As a result I look and feel thinner and younger than ever before.

As far as other things that have changed since I researched ageing, I now try to exercise every day, even if it's just a walk or stretching in front of the TV, and I am also religious about my cleansing routine, exfoliating regularly and using creams with active ingredients that will nourish my skin from the outside.

But what and when I eat still remains my most potent anti-ageing tool.

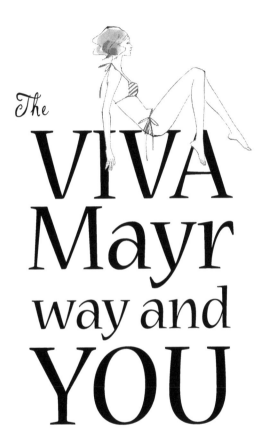

The

VIVA
Mayr
way and
YOU

You are about to discover:

How to assess your health and wellbeing,
from top to toe

How to ensure that the Viva Mayr way of
living becomes a habit that sticks

How to deal with weight-loss plateaus

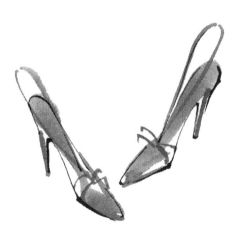

Today's Menu

Breakfast
Green tea, Viva vitality muesli (see page 272)

Lunch
Risotto patties with beetroot and asparagus, and blackberry crème (see pages 273–4)

Dinner
Spelt bread with vegetable spread, and potato and lovage soup (see page 274)

This is it, Day Fourteen. Well done! You've made it! By now you should be looking and feeling healthier, slimmer and more relaxed. You'll probably be sleeping better and have more energy than you've ever had before. It's very likely, too, that your tummy is less bloated and your blood sugar levels are much more stable. You probably haven't even noticed that you are eating far less than you used to! More importantly, perhaps, you will have adopted a lot of new habits that should have become second nature, like chewing properly.

Are you stuck?

If things haven't shifted dramatically, we need to work out why. I'm guessing that most of you bought this book to feel healthier but, also, to lose some weight. So the first thing to do is to ascertain whether or not that has happened. If you have been following the Viva Mayr approach religiously, there is absolutely no way that you won't be looking and feeling healthier and much slimmer (unless, of course, you've been supplementing with Krispy Kremes – or shortbread!).

If things haven't worked out the way you planned, take a look at the following short list of Viva Mayr essentials. If you aren't managing to stick to these, progress will be a little slower. Make an effort, now, to adjust your lifestyle to make them happen. It's worth it, I promise. Go back to the relevant sections of the book which deal with these 'essentials'; you'll find helpful tips for managing to live the Viva Mayr way in even the busiest household.

1 Chew, chew and chew again – aim for 30–40 chews for every mouthful you take.

2 Drink water *only* between meals; in fact, don't drink anything but teaspoonfuls of herbal tea when you are eating. But aim for a good two to three litres of water each day, which means sipping regularly between mealtimes.

3 Never eat raw after four. It's better to eat nothing than to upset your digestion by feeding your body raw foods too late.

4 Eat earlier in general – go for the six o'clock threshold, and, if possible, avoid eating anything after that time. If things don't exactly work out, eat a small, easily digestible snack in the evening rather than a huge meal.

5 Breakfast like a king; have a good-sized lunch, and then keep your dinner small and light.

6 Never eat when you are stressed, rushed or feeling upset. Wait until you are feeling calmer before sitting down to a meal.

7 Stop eating when you feel full – in fact, stop just before you 'think' you are full, to give your brain a chance to register that fact.

8 Exercise every day – some aerobic exercise is great, but even a little stretching is better than nothing.

9 Combine your foods so that you eat about twice as many alkaline foods (base foods) as you do acid foods. Create your own base powder and take base baths to encourage overall health and good digestion.

10 Bump up your intake of antioxidant-rich foods, such as brightly coloured fruit and vegetables and whole grains. Your skin – and your body – will love you for it! And you'll look and feel younger within a few short weeks.

Viva Mayr maintenance

So how do you maintain the Viva Mayr way of life, once you get back into the swing of things and are faced with more temptations and periods when you are so busy, you simply don't have time for yourself? How do you maintain your weight loss, and continue to feel energetic and healthy?

In terms of weight, it's important to remember that the Viva Mayr Diet is not a yo-you diet. It's a permanent eating plan, and the excess weight you lose will stay off. As Dr Stossier says, it's impossible to be healthy and overweight, and this diet ensures that we are about as healthy as it gets. If you haven't lost all the weight you hoped to, persevere. Slow weight loss is ideal, as it means that you are losing fat rather than just water and muscle.

In the real world, of course, there will be all sorts of occasions when it is impossible to live strictly by the rules. Someone might serve you a salad for dinner, or you may be on a business trip and have to eat in a rush before your next meeting. But you do have tools at your disposal to help to make these slips less damaging: chewing! Chewing can counter many ills, and no one can stop you from doing it. If you are eating salad too late for your body to cope with digesting it, then do as much of the digestive process in your mouth as you can. You can never chew enough. Similarly, if you are stressed and in a hurry but simply have to have something to eat, choose light meals, and chew them to death! It makes all the difference.

If you have to miss breakfast for whatever reason, eat a big lunch and try to re-establish your eating patterns the following day. Now that you have come this far, there is no need to let a minor blip ruin everything – even if you have had one too many shortbread biscuits or tequila slammers in a weak moment. Remember that the Viva Mayr way of eating and living is an investment in your future health and wellbeing. As well as keeping you thin, it will keep you healthy. Just think about all those diseases you are avoiding and how much better you feel – and will feel in the future.

Living the Viva Mayr life

The following guidelines will help you to be a Viva Mayr convert for life!

Turn food and eating into a priority in your life. Try to live to eat rather than eat to live. Really think about what you're eating, because it is going to have an effect both on how you feel in the short-term, and on your long-term health (not to mention looks!).

Chew without anything in your hands. It will slow you down, as you won't be rushing to take another bite.

Try to eat when you are relaxed. Don't focus on your mortgage statement, the crashing stock market or the latest terrorist attack when you are eating. You'll get stressed and you simply won't produce the saliva you need to begin the digestive process.

Train yourself to stop when it's enough. If you have that awful 'stuffed full' feeling, then you have eaten too much; try to eat less next time.

Use a small plate. This will ensure that your portions are smaller, and you will have the psychological advantage of having finished your plateful, which sends a message to your brain that you are full. If you are still hungry, by all means eat more. There are no hard-and-fast rules about portion size. As you become healthier, you will automatically learn to eat exactly what your body needs, rather than what your brain tells you it does!

Take smaller mouthfuls and *chew, chew, chew.* This is the single most important thing you can do, regardless of what and when you eat.

Don't drink with meals, as it dilutes saliva and reduces the capacity of your digestive system. Drink lots and lots in between meals instead, but stop 15 minutes before eating, and don't drink again until an hour after you've finished. What are the best drinks? Fresh, pure water, herbal teas, and fruit and vegetable juices are your best bets.

Recognise the signs that you haven't digested properly. If you crave something sweet after you've eaten, it could simply be habit; however, it could also be a sign that you have eaten so much that your body is asking for more energy. When we crave sweet things, it's often a signal that our cells aren't getting the energy they need, and the most likely cause of this is because digestion has slowed down, and nutrients are not being assimilated as they should. There is absolutely nothing wrong with the odd sweet treat, however, and there are plenty of healthy options available.

Don't be tempted to snack between meals, though. Our digestive systems need a rest between meals, to prepare themselves for the next onslaught! If you feel hungry, have a drink of juice, water or tea.

Give yourself time to eat. It is better to skip a meal entirely than to eat in a state of stress, or on the hoof.

Eat less in evenings. This is very difficult for cultural reasons, but it is essential for your health. If you can't manage it all the time, eat before six twice a week, and then build up to four times and eventually seven days. If you do have to go out to dinner late, eat as little as possible and chew everything to a liquidy pulp.

Give yourself time to digest. Don't exercise immediately after eating, or do anything too strenuous. Let your body use the energy for digestion instead.

Don't go into a supermarket when you are hungry.
This always results in buying too much – and often the wrong kinds of food.

Remember that we all eat far too much, so cut down on your portions.

Help your body to cope with stressful situations. If you are in a business meeting or at a dinner where you are focusing on other things apart from eating, make sure you choose an easily digestible meal and avoid alcohol.

Don't cook for people you don't like! It is well documented that eating well is not only contingent upon the food you choose but also the environment you eat it in. Eating with people you don't like is not going to be good for your digestive process. Eat in a stress-free situation.

Every meal should take you at least 30 minutes. Even if you are simply sitting at your desk with a sandwich, make the most of your meal. Savour your sandwich, and make it last. Look at your watch before you start and eek the sandwich out to make it last half an hour. You will never again experience that awful, exhausted feeling at the end of a meal.

Eat organic whenever possible. Organic food contains many more nutrients than conventionally farmed produce, so it's worth the extra money. What's more, it's full of vitality, which will be transmitted to you!

Never cook anything in a microwave. In fact, don't have a microwave in your kitchen at all. Not only do they remove nutrients from food, but they rob it of its vitality or 'life force'.

Always remember to live to your body's natural rhythms. Breakfast like a king when your digestive capacity is at its peak; lunch like a prince, when things are still going strong in the digestive department; then, dine like a pauper, when it all starts to slow down. You'll slow down as well, and experience a good night's sleep as a result. Eating little and early will leave you feeling fresh and invigorated every morning.

Never eat raw food after four. Your body won't be able to digest it properly, and you will experience discomfort and other symptoms as a result. What's more, you won't be able to digest or assimilate the nutrients your food contains, no matter how healthy that food might be.

Don't panic about missing a meal, especially dinner. This kind of involuntary fasting is not bad for you.

Break your bad habits – that is, eating or drinking anything that has zero nutritional value such as coca-cola, doughnuts or, um, shortbread. It really won't take long to break them and you will soon go off the very idea …

If you fall off the wagon, pick yourself up again. There is no need to give up just because you skipped breakfast once, or ate dinner at midnight. The Viva Mayr Diet is a life-long way of eating, and now that you have discovered it, you will always be able to incorporate it into your life.

Exercise is not an optional extra! Do something every day, even if it's just some stretching or going for a walk.

Make every little physical thing you do throughout the day work for you – for example, push yourself to bend, stretch and lift a little more when you are doing the housework, or increase your pace when walking up a hill.

When I first heard about Viva Mayr I thought, 'Oh, another diet.' Then I met Dr Stossier and realised that it is so much more – it is a way of life. Now that I have adopted it, I am a total addict and just can't imagine life without it. I even surprise myself with how hooked I am. Last night my husband ate an avocado for dinner. I ate some cheese and oatcakes. It didn't even occur to me to join him. For me, raw after four is no longer an option. Now I just have to convert the rest of my family.

I have managed to get them to slow down, at least. After almost a year of eating the Viva Mayr way I find watching someone wolf (just had to use that word one last time) down their food is positively painful. I think about all the damage they are doing to their insides and just want to tell them to stop, or rather CHEW!

I imagine I will carry on eating the Viva Mayr way for ever; that I will be chewing like a good 'un even when I no longer have my own teeth to do the job with. I am eternally grateful to Dr Stossier and his Viva Mayr team for teaching me how to eat. It is something so basic and simple and yet something it is so easy to get horribly wrong until you know the right way. Which if you have got this far you do. Now go forth and … chew.

In summary ...

- Viva Mayr is not just a diet, it's a way of life.

- It's perfectly possible to fall off the wagon and climb right back on without any significant dents in your progress.

- If you can't eat the right foods at the right time, you can redress the damage by chewing as long and hard as you can.

- You can make small adjustments to the way you live your life, working on a day to day basis, until you look and feel better than you ever have before. Because that's what Viva Mayr is all about – being the best you can be, and getting the very most you can out of life.

Case Study

Fiona, 58, Brighton

I went to the Viva Mayr clinic as a 50th birthday present to myself. I thought it would be impossible to carry on the diet once I got back to normal life, but at the same time I was really upset at the thought of just throwing away everything I had learned. So when I got back I made a real effort to incorporate the major rules.

Chewing was easy and so was raw before four – most of the time. The most difficult thing for me was not eating late. My husband doesn't get back from work until about half-past seven most nights, and we really enjoy eating together. It's a way of marking the end of the working day, and relaxing. So here is how I compromise: I have done away with the aperitif (apart from at weekends), so as soon as he's caught his breath we sit down to eat. I cook things that I know are easy to digest, like vegetable soups or baked potatoes, and I chew like mad. I give myself small portions, and one evening a week I do a mini-fast and have no dinner at all. The weight I lost all those years ago at the clinic has stayed off and I feel great. Better still, my husband has lost some excess weight as well, and he says he hasn't felt so well in years!

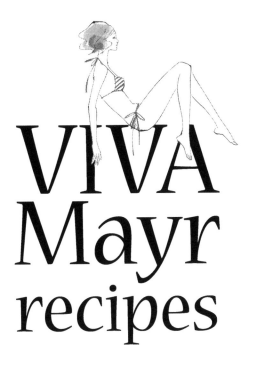

VIVA
Mayr
recipes

The meals recommended for the 14 days of your Viva Mayr diet have been designed as an integrated programme. They take account of all the Viva Mayr principles, such as easy digestibility, maintaining acid-base balance and avoiding uncooked vegetables in the evening.

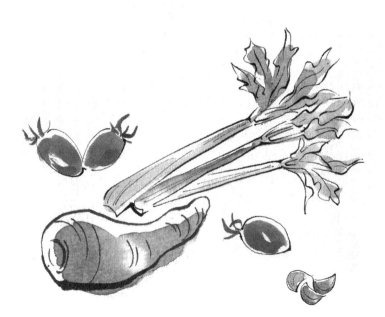

All recipes can be prepared in advance. Spreads and soups will keep in the fridge for two to three days. You can freeze freshly-baked Viva breads and rolls then take out whatever you require the next day to defrost overnight.

If you work in an office, simply prepare your lunches the night before and take them with you in a Tupperware-style box. The best way to reheat them is in a steamer. Please avoid using a microwave if at all possible. If you are unable to reheat your meal, it is far healthier to eat it cold than use a microwave, which will destroy all the precious vitamins, nutrients and minerals. *

If you go out to a restaurant during this period, that's not a problem. For lunch, choose a light, two-course meal, with a salad starter and a healthy main course, or a main course and a small dessert. For dinner, follow the food-combining rules so that your meal is easy to digest: fish, meat, pasta, potatoes or rice should be served with vegetables but not with each other, so no fish and chips or meat with rice. And remember to chew!

I hope you enjoy our recipes and the introduction to our healthy style of cuisine.

* The Journal of the Science of Food and Agriculture, Issue no. 44 (2003).

Day One

Fruit muesli *with* nuts

Serves Two

80g soft, fresh goat's or sheep's cheese (unsalted)

100g fresh, ripe fruits of the season

15g walnuts

15g almonds

2 tbsp whole linseeds (flaxseeds)

1 tsp honey

2–3 tbsp unsweetened soya milk

Lemon or orange juice (to taste)

3 tbsp oil (choose from linseed/flaxseed or hemp)

In a coffee-bean grinder or food processor, grind together the walnuts, almonds and linseeds until roughly chopped.

Place in a glass bowl, and stir in the cheese, honey and soya milk. Season with lemon or orange juice to taste.

Peel and dice fruit (leaving berries whole).

Distribute the creamy mixture equally into two bowls, and sprinkle with the fruit. Drizzle with oil and serve immediately.

Vegetable salad *with* chicken strips

Serves Four

Coconut oil

2 pinches of rock salt

4 chicken breasts, skinless and boneless

1 stalk rosemary, chopped

4 tbsp oil (such as, hemp, olive or sunflower)

2 tbsp cider vinegar

500g mixed salad leaves

2 tomatoes, diced

1 carrot, peeled and diced

4 radishes, diced

1 kohlrabi, cut into strips

Fresh herbs, such as basil, thyme, marjoram or parsley, to garnish

Heat a little coconut oil in a frying pan. Season the chicken breasts with one pinch of salt, sprinkle with rosemary, and fry for 8 to 10 minutes, or until the chicken is lightly browned and cooked through. Cut the chicken into strips and set to one side.

Blend together the oil, cider vinegar and the final pinch of rock salt. Mix together your salad leaves and vegetables, and dress with the oil and vinegar dressing. Serve on a platter with the chicken on top. Garnish with fresh herbs of your choice.

Fresh berry cream

Serves Four

120g fresh, soft goat's or sheep's cheese
100g fresh berry purée
2 tbsp honey

250ml fresh cream, whipped
4 fresh mint leaves

Blend together the cheese, berry purée (reserving about 20ml for later) and honey. Fold in the whipped cream, and decant into four individual glasses. Spoon a teaspoon of berry purée over the top of each of the berry creams, and then garnish with a mint leaf. Serve immediately.

Note: You can make your own fresh berry purée by Whizzing berries in a liquidiser or food processor until smooth. Strain through a sieve to remove any seeds or pips. Alternatively, choose a ready-prepared purée with no added sugar.

Soft polenta *with* steamed vegetables and herbs

Serves Four

500ml water or vegetable stock
200g very fine polenta
20g butter
Rock salt, to taste
100g broccoli, cubed

100g fennel, cubed
100g carrots, cubed
100g courgettes, cubed
100g kohlrabi, cubed
Fresh marjoram or basil leaves, to garnish

In a saucepan, bring the water or vegetable stock to the boil, and stir in the polenta. Add the butter and sea salt, and continue cooking for a few more minutes. Remove the polenta from the heat, cover the saucepan and leave to sit for 20 minutes, until all of the liquid is absorbed and the polenta is light and fluffy.

Next, boil the vegetables briefly in a little salted water, or steam for a few minutes.

Place the polenta on plates, and arrange vegetables over top. Sprinkle with marjoram or basil, and serve.

Day Two

Mixed vegetable sticks

Serves Two

50g carrots, peeled and cut into batons

50g celery stalks, cut into batons

50g spring onions or fresh radish, cut into small strips

50g tomatoes, quartered

Place the vegetables on a platter, and serve with Viva spread, or any other herbal spread (see page 279).

Leafy salad *with* walnuts, apples and linseed dressing

Serves Four

400g mixed salad leaves

2 apples, cored and quartered

50g whole walnuts

4 tbsp linseed oil

2 tbsp freshly squeezed lime juice

2-3 leaves of fresh basil

1 tbsp sour cream

A pinch of rock salt

1 punnet garden cress

Wash salad leaves thoroughly and spin dry. Add the apples and walnuts and set to one side.

In a liquidiser, blend together the linseed oil, lime juice, basil, sour cream and salt until smooth and creamy.

Arrange the salad on glass plates and sprinkle with dressing. Top with garden cress, and serve.

Potato and vegetable gratin *with* spinach sauce

Serves Four

1kg waxy potatoes, washed, peeled
   and cut into very thin slices
100g carrots, washed and grated
100g courgettes, washed and grated
100g celeriac, washed and grated
250ml double cream
Fresh herbs, such as basil, thyme
   and parsley, finely chopped.

1 nutmeg, grated
Pinch of rock salt
Olive oil
500ml vegetable stock or water
300g fresh spinach, washed
A pinch of rock salt
A pinch of grated nutmeg

Preheat the oven to 175°C, 325°F, Gas mark 3.

Blend together the sliced potato and grated vegetables, and stir in the cream. Season with the fresh herbs, nutmeg and rock salt.

Next, grease an oven-proof baking dish with olive oil, and pour in the potato and vegetable mixture. Bake for about 40 minutes.

While it's cooking, bring your water or vegetable stock to the boil, and add the spinach. Boil for one minute, and then liquidise the spinach with the stock. Season to taste with rock salt and ground nutmeg. If desired, add fresh herbs to add more flavour, such as parsley, coriander and dill.

When the gratin is cooked, and nicely browned, remove it from the oven and serve immediately with warm spinach sauce.

Poached trout *with* vegetables and lemongrass

Serves Four

500ml organic vegetable stock or water

A small bunch of fresh basil or parsley, finely chopped

1 stalk lemongrass, chopped

A pinch of rock salt

4 fresh trout fillets (you can substitute salmon, if you wish)

100g carrots, cut into 2mm semi-circles

100g celery, cut into 2mm semi-circles

100g parsnip, cut into 2mm semi-circles

100g courgettes, cut into 2mm semi-circles

Lemongrass and fresh herbs, chopped, to garnish

In a shallow pan, bring the stock or water to a boil, and stir in the freshly chopped herbs, lemongrass and salt.

Next, preheat a non-stick frying pan and add a few drops of olive oil. When hot, add the vegetables and stir-fry them for a few minutes.

Add the fish fillets to the herby stock and poach for a few minutes. Remove them from the poaching liquid, and set them to one side. Cover. Pour the stock over the stir-fried vegetables, and simmer until tender. Drain.

Arrange the vegetables on a plate, and top with your fish. Sprinkle with fresh lemongrass and herbs, and serve.

Day Three

Courgette soup

Serves Four

1 litre organic vegetable stock or water
100g potatoes, peeled and chopped
300g courgettes, peeled and chopped
A pinch of rock salt
A small bunch of fresh parsley, finely chopped
4 tsp oil (linseed, hemp or olive)

In a large pan, bring the water or stock to the boil, and add the potatoes. Simmer for 8 to 10 minutes, and then add the courgettes. Continue boiling for a further 4 minutes.

Remove from the heat and use a blender or liquidiser to purée until smooth. Stir in the parsley and salt to taste, and serve in bowls with a little oil drizzled over the top.

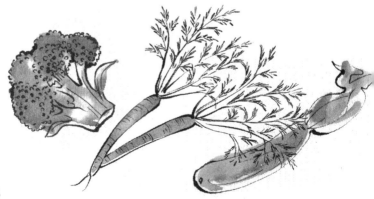

Grilled chicken on hash-browned potatoes and vegetables with fresh herb oil

Serves Four

200g waxy potatoes
100g kohlrabi, peeled and sliced
110g carrots, peeled and sliced
100g celery, peeled and sliced
1 tbsp coconut oil
4 chicken breasts, skinless and boneless

6 tbsp extra-virgin olive oil
1 bunch each of fresh basil and parsley, chopped
2 tbsp fresh rosemary and thyme, chopped
Pinch of rock salt

Bring a large pot of water to the boil, and add the potatoes, cooking them in their skins until tender. When they are cool enough to touch, peel and cut into slices. Next, steam or blanch the remaining vegetables for a few minutes.

Heat a little coconut oil in a frying pan, and add the potatoes and vegetables. Fry, turning often, until brown and slightly crispy.

As the hash browns are cooking, heat a little more coconut oil in another frying pan, until hot, and gently fry the chicken until lightly browned, turning frequently.

As the chicken and hash browns are cooking, place the olive oil and the fresh herbs in a food processor and purée until smooth.

Season hash-browned potatoes and vegetables with the rosemary, thyme and sea salt, and place the chicken on top. Drizzle with fresh herb oil, and serve immediately.

Buckwheat blinis *with* vegetable cubes

Serves Four

400g potatoes
4 eggs, beaten
100g very fine buckwheat flour
125ml cream
A pinch of rock salt
A pinch of grated nutmeg
2 tbsp olive oil

1 courgette, cubed
1 aubergine, cubed
1 kohlrabi, cubed
1 celery stalk, cubed
125ml organic vegetable stock
A handful of fresh herbs (basil, parsley
    and coriander, for example), chopped

In a large pan, bring water to the boil and add the potatoes. Cook them in their skins until tender (about 8 to 10 minutes). Drain and cool slightly. Remove the skin, and press the potatoes through a ricer, or knead with your hands until soft. Place in a bowl and stir in the eggs, flour, cream, salt and nutmeg. Beat with a whisk. If the liquid is too runny, add a little more flour to give it more body. Form small pancakes or patties with your hands and set to one side.

Next, add a tablespoon of olive to a wok, and heat until hot. Add the vegetables, and stir for a few moments. Then add the vegetable stock and simmer until the vegetables are crisp, but tender.

As you are cooking the vegetables, slowly heat a frying pan with a few drops of olive oil, and cook the blinis for about 2 minutes per side.

When the vegetables are cooked, stir in the fresh herbs and season with rock salt. Spoon over the blinis and serve immediately.

Pomegranate juice

Drink a small glass of good-quality pomegranate juice, spoonful by spoonful, to encourage you to learn to chew.

Day Four

Viva muesli *with* soft cheese and fresh fruit

Serves Two

120g fresh, seasonal fruit, diced
100g soft, fresh goat's or sheep's cheese
3 tbsp linseed oil

30g walnuts, to garnish
Mint leaves, to garnish

Place the diced fruit in a glass bowl. Mix together the cheese and oil until creamy, adding a few tbsp of water or oil if it seems too dry. Pour over the diced fruit, and garnish with walnuts and mint leaves.

Broccoli soup

Serves Four

1 litre water or organic vegetable stock
300g broccoli, washed and cut into
    small pieces
100g potatoes, peeled and chopped

Rock salt, to taste
Ground nutmeg, to taste
2 tbsp extra-virgin nut oil

Bring the water or vegetable stock to the boil in a large pan, and add the potatoes. Cook for 5 minutes, and then add the broccoli and simmer for seven more. Remove from the heat, and purée in a food processor or blender, until smooth. Season with nutmeg and rock salt, and return to the heat. When piping hot, serve immediately, drizzled with a few drops of nut oil.

Wild salmon *with* spinach and carrot mash

Serves Four

200g carrots, peeled and chopped
A pinch of rock salt
1 stalk lemongrass
A pinch of freshly grated ginger
250ml organic vegetable stock
4, 120g fillets of organic wild salmon

½ tbsp butter
400g fresh organic spinach, washed
   with hard stalks removed
Grated nutmeg, to taste
A handful of fresh basil, chopped
6 tbsp olive oil

Place the carrots in a small saucepan, and simmer, covered, for 5 to 7 minutes, or until tender. Remove from the heat and mash or blend in a food processor until smooth. Add lemongrass and fresh ginger, and season with rock salt. Set to one side, and cover to keep warm.

In a frying pan or wok, heat the vegetable stock. Salt the salmon fillets with a little rock salt, and place in the stock. Cover and simmer for a few minutes, until tender.

While the fish is cooking, melt the butter in a saucepan, and cook the spinach for 1 to 2 minutes, or until tender. Season with rock salt and a grating of nutmeg.

In a food processor or blender, mix together the chopped basil and olive oil until it becomes a glorious green colour. Add a little rock salt to taste.

Place a bed of spinach on each plate, topped with the carrot mash and the fish. Sprinkle with basil oil, and serve immediately.

Note: any extra oil can be stored in the fridge for a few days, stored in a glass bottle or jar.

Baked potato *with* fresh herb dip

Serves Four

4 large baking potatoes
Olive oil
4 stalks rosemary
100g sour cream
4 tbsp chopped herbs, such as parsley, lovage, basil, chervil and/or coriander
1 tbsp olive oil
A pinch of rock salt

Preheat the oven to 175°C, 325°F, gas mark 3.

Wash the potatoes, prick them, and brush with a little olive oil. Wrap in aluminium foil, tucking a stalk of rosemary in each foil packet. Bake for 40 to 50 minutes, or until tender.

Blend together the sour cream, herbs, oil and salt until smooth.

Open the potatoes, and fill with fresh herb dip. Serve immediately.

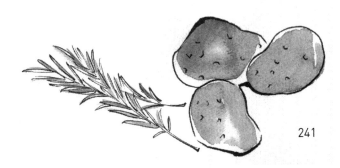

Day Five

Oat porridge *with* fresh fruit and linseed oil

Serves Two

350ml water
130g ground oat flakes
A pinch of rock salt
2 tbsp linseed oil
Fresh, seasonal fruit, chopped
2 tsp honey or maple syrup
Linseed oil, to taste

In a saucepan, bring the water to a boil, and stir in the oat flakes. When the oats are boiling, remove from the heat and cover for 3 to 5 minutes.

Next, stir the chopped fruit into the porridge, and spoon into two bowls. Drizzle with honey or maple syrup, and then add a little linseed oil. Serve immediately.

Vegetable risotto *with* olives, basil and Parmesan

Serves Four

1 tbsp olive oil
2 shallots, finely chopped
300g risotto rice, rinsed under cold water
150ml tomato juice
1 litre vegetable stock, or water
300g mixed vegetables such as carrot, courgette, fennel, cut into small cubes
16 green or black olives
About 3 pinches of rock salt
1 tbsp finely chopped fresh basil
4 tbsp freshly grated Parmesan

Heat the olive oil in a saucepan, add the shallots and slowly sweat, until they are translucent. Add the rice and turn up the heat. Keep stirring until the rice starts to sweat, being careful not to brown the shallots or the rice. Add the tomato juice and stir. Slowly add the vegetable stock or water, ladle by ladle, stirring constantly. Bring to the boil and reduce the heat. When the rice is almost cooked (after about 10 minutes) gradually stir in the diced vegetables and green olives and season with the rock salt. It should be ready in another 5 minutes. To serve, sprinkle with the fresh basil and Parmesan.

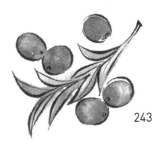

Rice burgers *with* beetroot ragout and asparagus

Serves Four

500g soft, cooked risotto rice

125ml single cream

2 eggs, beaten

A pinch of rock salt

A pinch of grated nutmeg

3 tbsp chopped parsley

1kg fresh beetroot, washed and peeled

1 cinnamon stick

1 tsp cloves

1 tbsp potato flour

400g asparagus

1 tbsp butter

Freshly chopped herbs, to garnish

Mix together the risotto rice, cream, eggs, salt, nutmeg and parsley. Form into small burgers.

Heat a frying pan with a few drops of coconut oil, and fry the burgers, turning frequently, until golden brown.

Dice half of the beetroot, and place the other half into a juicer. Blend the diced beetroot and the beetroot juice, and place in a small saucepan. Add a little rock salt, a cinnamon stick and the cloves, and simmer until soft.

In a small bowl, blend together the potato flour with a little cold water. Add to the beetroot, and cook gently until thickened.

In another pan, bring some slightly salted water to the boil, and cook the asparagus until softened. Toss with a little butter.

Arrange the beetroot ragout in the centre of each plate, and position the rice burgers on top. Decorate the plate's rim with green asparagus and garnish with fresh herbs.

Day Six

Linseed yoghurt *with* papaya and maple syrup

Serves Two

15g walnuts
2 tbsp linseeds
200g live yoghurt
  (cow's, sheep's or goat's)

2 tbsp linseed oil
1 tsp maple syrup
Freshly squeezed lemon or orange juice,
  to taste
100g papaya, peeled and diced

In a coffee-bean grinder or food-processor, coarsely chop the walnuts and linseeds. Place in a glass bowl, and add the yoghurt, linseed oil and maple syrup. Season to taste with a few drops of lemon or orange juice.

Decant into two bowls, and generously cover with the papaya. Serve immediately.

Fruity sprouted salad *with* linseeds

Serves Four

200g soya bean sprouts
4 tbsp mixed sprouts, such as
  fenugreek, alfalfa, mung bean
  or radish
1 carrot, peeled and finely sliced
1 apple, cored, and finely sliced
1 orange, peeled and finely sliced

1 pomegranate, halved seeds removed
1 mango, peeled and finely sliced
2 tbsp virgin linseed oil,
Juice of 1 lime
A handful of fresh basil leaves
Rock salt, to taste
2 tbsp linseeds

Wash and drain the sprouts, and place them on a large plate.

Mix together the carrot, apple, orange, pomegranate seeds and mango. Place on top of the sprouts, and sprinkle with linseed oil and lime juice. Scatter with fresh basil and linseeds, and serve immediately.

Celeriac *with* slices of turkey ham, vegetables and fresh herb cream

Serves Four

2 fresh celeriac, cut into thick slices
A handful of fresh herbs
Rock salt, to taste
2 medium potatoes, peeled and chopped
Fresh herbs, such as basil, lovage, parsley or chervil, finely chopped

2 tbsp olive oil
An assortment of mixed vegetables, such as courgettes, tomatoes, aubergines, kohlrabi and fennel, diced
8 slices of turkey ham

Preheat the oven to 180°C, 350°F, gas mark 4.

Wrap each slice of celeriac in a square of aluminium foil, adding a sprinkling of fresh herbs and rock salt before sealing. Roast for 15–18 minutes.

While it's cooking, make the herb cream. Add the potatoes to a pot of salted water, and cook until tender. Remove from the heat, and mix the potatoes in a food processor with the chopped herbs and rock salt, until smooth. The herb cream should be a verdant, green colour.

Next heat the olive oil in a frying pan, and add the diced vegetables. Lightly fry until just tender.

Place a slice of celeriac on the plate, cover with the diced vegetable mixture, top that with a small slice of turkey ham, and then another slice of celeriac, and so on …

Serve with fresh herb cream.

Asian-style vegetables *with* lemongrass and herbs

Serves Four

1 tsp warm-pressed olive oil
3 tbsp vegetable stock
100g carrots, peeled and cut into
   thin strips
100g organic celeriac, peeled and cut
   into thin strips
100g courgettes, peeled and cut into
   thin strips

50g fresh fennel, cut into thin strips
100g sprouting soya beans
1 stalk lemongrass, chopped
2 tbsp organic soya sauce
2 tbsp fresh herbs, such as basil or
   parsley, chopped

Heat the olive oil in a wok or heavy-bottomed pan, and add the vegetable stock and sliced vegetables. Stir in the soya bean sprouts, and cook until the juices have evaporated, tossing constantly. Sprinkle with fresh herbs, and serve immediately.

Day Seven

Hummus

400g dried chickpeas
2 tbsp extra-virgin olive oil
3 tbsp lemon juice
2 pinches of rock salt

Soak the chickpeas in plenty of cold water for at least 24 hours. Rinse under cold water, and then boil them in slightly salted water for about 20 minutes.

Drain, and place in a food processor or liquidiser with the olive oil, lemon juice and salt. Blend together until smooth, adding a little water if it is too thick.

Serve with vegetable sticks (see page 233).

Note: You can use ready-made hummus from a good health-food shop, if necessary.

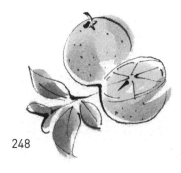

Rocket salad *with* smoked salmon and horseradish

Serves Four

200g fresh rocket
1 tbsp cold-pressed extra-virgin olive oil
1 tsp balsamic vinegar
A pinch of rock salt
8 slices of smoked salmon
1 tbsp freshly grated horseradish (or good-quality ready-made horseradish sauce)

Mix the rocket in a glass bowl with the olive oil and balsamic vinegar, then season to taste with a little rock salt. To serve, arrange the dressed rocket on individual plates, place the smoked salmon slices on top and sprinkle with the fresh horseradish (or the ready-made sauce).

Buckwheat crêpes *with* parsnips and chervil cream

Serves Four

250ml milk
125g finely ground buckwheat flour
2 eggs, lightly beaten
A pinch of rock salt
1 tbsp parsley, finely chopped
2 medium potatoes, peeled and cubed

A small bunch of fresh chervil
Rock salt, to taste
300g fresh parsnips, peeled and cubed
A pinch of freshly ground nutmeg
Fresh herbs, chopped, to garnish

Mix together all of the ingredients in a food processor, or a mixer, until smooth.

Gently heat some coconut oil in a frying pan, and add a little of the batter to the centre of the hot pan, spreading it quickly with the back of a spoon so that it is thinly spread. Cook for about 30 seconds on one side, and then flip and cook on the other side. Continue until you have used all of your batter.

Make the chervil cream by boiling the potatoes in lightly salted water, until tender, and then puréeing in a food processor or liquidiser with the chervil and some salt. Spread this cream on four individual plates and set to one side.

Next, add the parsnips to a saucepan of boiling, lightly salted water and cook until tender. Remove from the heat, and purée half of the parsnip cubes in a food processor or liquidiser. Stir into the remaining cubes, and season with rock salt and nutmeg. The purée should be thick and a bit dry. If it is too liquid, reheat, simmering slowly until the water evaporates.

Spread the crêpes with the parsnip mixture, and roll them up. Cut each crêpe into 3, and place on the chervil cream. Garnish with fresh herbs, and serve immediately.

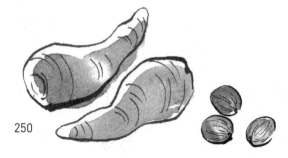

Tarragon tofu burgers
with fresh vegetable stew

Serves Four

300g silken tofu

2 eggs, beaten

2 tbsp soya flour

A small bunch of organic tarragon, finely chopped

A pinch of rock salt

Coconut oil

250ml vegetable juice, such as carrot, fennel or celeriac

150g carrots, peeled and cut into small pieces

150g courgettes, peeled and cut into small pieces

150g broccoli, cut into florettes

150g fennel, cut into cubes

1 tbsp potato flour

A handful of fresh herbs, such as parsley, coriander, basil or dill, finely chopped

In a food processor or blender, mix together the tofu, eggs, soya flour, tarragon and salt, until you have a lovely cream. Remove from the processor, and form into patties that are approximately 50g.

Heat the coconut oil in a frying pan, and cook the patties, turning regularly, until golden brown.

Next, bring the vegetable juice to the boil in a small pan and add the vegetables, cooking until tender. Mix together the potato flour with a little water, and stir into the stew. Season to taste, and add a handful of fresh herbs.

Ladle the stew on to the plates, and serve with the tofu burgers on top, strewn with a garnish of fresh herbs.

Day Eight

Avocado, tomato and mozzarella *with* basil pesto

Serves Two

2 tbsp extra-virgin olive oil
A handful of fresh basil, very finely
  chopped
1 or 2 ripe avocados, peeled and sliced

1 or 2 large, ripe tomatoes, cut into
  quarters
2 balls of mozzarella, sliced

Make the basil pesto by blending together the olive oil and fresh basil.

Next, arrange the avocados, tomatoes and mozzarella on a plate, and sprinkle with pesto. Serve immediately.

Carrot *and* ginger soup

Serves Four

300g carrots, washed and chopped
100g potatoes, washed and chopped
750ml water or vegetable stock

A small ginger root, grated
A pinch of rock salt

Juice about a third of the carrots, and set to one side. In a saucepan heat the water or vegetable stock, and add the remaining carrots and potatoes. Cook until tender, and remove from the heat.

In a food processor or liquidiser, blend the carrots and potatoes with the ginger and the water or stock, until smooth. Stir in the carrot juice, and season with salt to taste. Gently reheat (avoiding bringing the soup to a boil), and serve immediately.

Turkey and rosemary skewers
with sautéed fennel and courgettes,
and truffle oil

Serves Four

2 large organic turkey breasts, skinless and boneless, each cut into 6 equal pieces
4 long stalks rosemary
Coconut oil
Fresh fennel, cut into fine strips
4 small courgettes, cut into fine semi-circles
Fresh herbs, such as basil, chervil, parsley, coriander or tarragon, finely chopped
Rock salt, to taste
Truffle oil (optional)

Spear three pieces of the turkey on each rosemary stalk. Season lightly with salt. Heat some coconut oil in a heavy-bottomed pan, and gently fry the turkey at medium heat, until lightly browned and cooked through.

Next, add a little coconut oil to a wok, and, when hot, add the vegetables and cook for about 3 to 4 minutes. Season with rock salt and fresh herbs.

To serve, place the vegetables in the centre of the plate, and top with a turkey skewer. Decorate with fresh herb sprigs and, if desired, a few drops of truffle oil.

Potato cakes *with* cottage cheese and linseed oil

Serves Four

600g organic waxy potatoes, grated
2 egg yolks, beaten
A pinch of grated nutmeg
A pinch of rock salt
1 tbsp olive oil

200g cottage cheese
1 tbsp linseed oil
A handful of fresh herbs, chopped,
   to garnish

Dry the grated potatoes in some kitchen towel, and press out all the water. Mix together with the egg yolks, nutmeg and rock salt. Form the mixture into patties.

Heat the olive oil in a frying pan until hot, and fry the potato cakes on both sides, until golden brown, and crispy. Place on a piece of kitchen towel to absorb any excess oil.

Place the potato cakes on a plate, and add a dollop of cottage cheese on top of each. Sprinkle with linseed oil and fresh herbs, and serve.

Day Nine

Freshly pressed fruit *and* vegetable juice

Serves Two

2 large apples, washed and diced
2 oranges, peeled and diced
2 grapefruit, peeled and diced

2 carrots, peeled and diced
½ celeriac, washed and diced
1–2 tbsp olive oil (or linseed or hemp)

Feed all of the ingredients into a juicer. Immediately pour into tall glasses, and add a few drops of oil. Serve at once.

Root vegetable soup

Serves Four

1 tsp coconut oil
50g shallots, chopped
150g potatoes, peeled and chopped
50g carrots, peeled and chopped
50g parsnips, peeled and chopped

5g turnips, peeled and chopped
50g celery, chopped
1 litre water
A pinch of rock salt
150ml fresh single cream

Slowly heat the coconut oil in a shallow saucepan, and then gently sweat the shallots over low heat, until soft but not brown. Add the chopped potatoes and vegetables, along with the water. Stir and simmer until tender, and then remove from the heat. Stir in the fresh cream, and blend in a liquidiser or food processor until smooth. Season to taste, and reheat gently to serve.

Millet casserole *with* broccoli purée

Serves Four

150g millet, washed

250g celeriac (or other root vegetables), washed and cubed

2 eggs yolks, beaten

A handful of fresh basil

A handful of fresh parsley

A pinch of grated nutmeg

A pinch of rock salt

2 egg whites, whipped to soft peaks

350g broccoli, washed and chopped

Preheat the oven to 170°C, 325°F, gas mark 3.

Simmer the millet in a little water until tender, and then drain, but do not rinse.

Next, cook the celeriac in a little water until tender, and remove from the heat. In a food processor or liquidiser, blend together the millet and celeriac. Add the egg yolks, salt, basil, parsley and nutmeg, and season with salt.

Gently fold the beaten egg whites into the millet mixture. Grease an oven-proof casserole dish, and fill with the mixture. Bake for 25 minutes.

While the millet casserole is cooking, boil the broccoli in a small saucepan with a little water, until tender. Blend in a food processor until smooth. If the sauce is too thick, add a little more water. Season with rock salt.

To serve, slice the millet casserole and serve on a plate, decorated with broccoli purée.

Vegetable terrine *with* fresh herb | and linseed cheese

Serves Four

300g broccoli, washed and cut into small pieces

500g celeriac, peeled and cut into small pieces

400g carrots, peeled and cut into small pieces

3 eggs

750ml vegetable stock or fresh cream

A pinch of rock salt

A good grating of fresh ginger

100g fresh, soft goat's or sheep's cheese

A handful of fresh herbs, such as basil, parsley or chervil, finely chopped

2 tbsp linseed oil

Preheat the oven to 170°C, 325°F, gas mark 3.

Steam or boil the vegetables separately, until tender. Next, in a food processor, blend the broccoli with one egg, and a third of the stock or cream, until smooth. Season with rock salt. Do the same with the celeriac. When you come to the carrots, blend with the ginger.

You will be left with three different vegetable purées.

Now, make the herb cheese by blending together the soft cheese with the fresh herbs and linseed oil.

Layer the purées in tall glasses, and top them with fresh herb cheese. Place the glasses in a bain marie, and simmer in the oven for 25 minutes.

Cover a plate with a napkin, place a glass of terrine on top, and drape with fresh herbs before serving.

Day Ten

Millet Porridge *with* dried fruit and linseed oil

Serves Two

350ml water
A pinch of rock salt
130g finely ground millet flakes

A handful of dried fruit, such as prune,
   sultanas, raisins and apricots, chopped
2 tsp honey or maple syrup
2 tbsp virgin linseed oil

In a saucepan, bring the water to a boil and stir in the millet flakes. When they begin to boil, remove the pan from the heat, cover, and leave to rest for 5 to 6 minutes. If you like your porridge runnier, add a little more water.

Stir the dried fruit into your porridge, and sweeten with honey or maple syrup. Drizzle the linseed oil over top, and serve instantly.

Carrot and beetroot salad *with* fresh lemon and coriander

Serves Four

200g carrots, peeled and grated
200g celeriac, peeled and grated
200g beetroot, peeled and grated
A small bunch of fresh coriander,
   coarsely chopped
2 tbsp linseed oil

2 tbsp fresh lemon juice
2 tbsp walnuts, coarsely chopped
¼ tsp ginger root, freshly grated
A pinch of rock salt
1 orange, peeled and segmented

Grate the carrots, celeriac and beetroot. In a large bowl, mix together the grated vegetables, coriander, linseed oil, fresh lemon juice, walnuts and ginger. Mix thoroughly, and season to taste.

Arrange on a plate, and place the orange segments on top. Serve immediately.

Lamb loin with celeriac and broccoli

Serves Four

400g lamb loin cut into 4 pieces	1 medium-sized celeriac, peeled
2 pinches of mixed fresh herbs,	and chopped
such as fresh thyme, coriander	A pinch of rock salt
and rosemary, finely chopped	½ tsp truffle oil
A few drops of coconut oil	300g broccoli

Preheat oven to 170°C, 325°F, gas mark 3.

Rub the lamb with three-quarters of the herb mixture. Heat a few drops of coconut oil in a frying pan. Add the fillets and cook over a medium heat to brown the outsides. Remove to a roasting tin and cook in the oven for 7 minutes, then take them out of the oven and let them stand.

Steam the celeriac in a shallow saucepan, covered with a lid, until tender. Blend to a purée and season with rock salt and a few drops of truffle oil.

Cut the broccoli into small florets and steam for 8 minutes.

Halve the lamb fillets and place on a hot plate. Add some celeriac purée and serve with broccoli florets. Sprinkle with the leftover fresh herbs and the rest of the truffle oil.

Potato and sesame-seed patties
with olive cream, courgettes
and oven-roasted tomatoes

Serves Four

720g waxy potatoes
2 egg yolks, lightly beaten
A handful of fresh herbs, such as basil,
   parsley and lovage, finely chopped
A pinch of rock salt
A pinch of ground nutmeg
100g sesame seeds

1 tbsp olive oil
2 medium potatoes, cooked
8 black or green olives, pitted
125ml water or organic vegetable stock
200g cherry tomatoes
2 medium courgettes, sliced

In a large pan of salted water, boil the potatoes in the skin until tender. When they are cool, peel them and press them through a ricer or a sieve.

In a good-sized bowl, blend together the potato, eggs, herbs, salt and nutmeg. Form into 8 patties, approximately 90g each, and then roll in the sesame seeds.

Next, preheat the oven to 180°C, 175°F, gas mark 4, to roast your tomatoes.

Heat the olive oil in a frying pan, and cook the patties on both sides, until golden brown. Keep them in a warm place until you are ready to serve.

When the oven's hot, place the tomatoes on a baking tray, and roast for 10 minutes.

Add the courgettes and a little vegetable stock to a frying pan, and simmer until tender.

Next make the olive cream. Simply reheat the cooked potatoes in the water or stock, add the olives, and boil for a minute. Remove from the heat, and blend in a food processor or liquidiser, until smooth. Season to taste.

Serve the patties with the courgettes and tomatoes on the side, and a good dollop of olive cream on top.

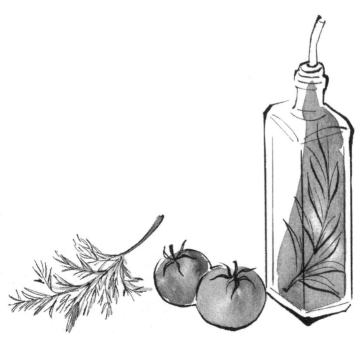

Day Eleven

Vegetable omelette *with* fresh herbs

Serves Two

Coconut oil (or olive oil)
100g seasonal mixed vegetables of your choice, peeled and finely sliced
4 eggs, beaten
Fresh herbs, such as coriander, basil or parsley, finely chopped
A pinch of rock salt

Heat a little coconut (or olive) oil in a pan, and add the vegetables. Let them sweat for about a minute, and then stir in the eggs and the fresh herbs. Whisk them continuously as the eggs begin to cook, and then let them cook through. Season to taste. Fold into half or thirds, and serve immediately.

Bowl of fresh salad

Serves Four

2 tbsp linseed oil
2 tbsp cider vinegar
A pinch of rock salt
500g mixed lettuce leaves, washed and shredded
Fresh herbs like basil and parsley, coarsely chopped

Blend together the oil, vinegar and salt, and put to one side.

Place the lettuce in a bowl, and drizzle with the dressing. Sprinkle with fresh herbs and serve.

Amaranth and vegetable curry

150g amaranth seeds
4–5 tbsp water or vegetable stock
250g fresh mixed vegetables, such as carrots, celeriac and courgettes,
   peeled and chopped into small pieces
1 tsp mild organic curry paste
1 tbsp olive oil
2–3 tbsp fresh herbs, such as basil and parsley, finely chopped
A pinch of rock salt

Rinse the amaranth seeds in warm water. Add to a saucepan of
boiling water. Cover and simmer for 12 to 15 minutes. Drain and
rinse with cold water.

Heat the water or vegetable stock, and steam the vegetables for 3
to 5 minutes. Reduce the heat, and simmer until most of the liquid
has been absorbed. Add the curry paste, olive oil and herbs, and
stir well.

Add the cooked amaranth seeds, and warm through. Season to
taste with rock salt, and serve warm.

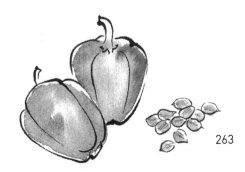

Potato blinis
with vegetable purée
and char caviar

Serves Four

320g potatoes, washed
100ml fresh cream
3 eggs, beaten
50g potato flour
A pinch of rock salt
A pinch of grated nutmeg
1 tsp coconut oil
250g celeriac, pumpkin or parsnip, peeled and chopped
1 tsp olive or linseed oil
A handful of fresh mixed herbs, such as parsley, basil, coriander or thyme, finely chopped
4 tablespoons char caviar

In a large saucepan, boil the potatoes in their skins until tender. Cool, and then peel and press through a potato ricer or sieve. Whisk in the cream, eggs, potato flour, salt and nutmeg.

Form the blinis, using a tablespoon. Heat the coconut oil in a frying pan, and drop in the blinis, cooking on both sides (about 4 to 5 minutes) until golden brown. Put the blinis in a warm place until required.

Next, boil the vegetables until tender. Season to taste, and blend in a food processor or liquidiser until smooth. Stir in the oil, and season with fresh herbs.

To serve, arrange the blinis on the plate, and spoon the vegetable purée into the centre. Place a teaspoon of char caviar on each, and serve.

Day Twelve

Papaya and banana salad, *with* cinnamon yoghurt and almond purée

Serves Two

200g almonds (peeled or unpeeled)
100ml water
3 tbsp almond or walnut oil
125ml live yoghurt (sheep's, goat's, soya or cow's milk)
A pinch of ground cinnamon
1 ripe papaya, peeled and chopped into small pieces
1 banana, peeled and chopped into small pieces

Place the almonds, water and oil in a food processor or liquidiser, and blend until creamy. Add a little water if the purée is too dry.

Next mix together the yoghurt and the cinnamon.

Place the yoghurt on a plate, and add a generous layer of banana and papaya on top. Add a dollop of almond purée and serve immediately.

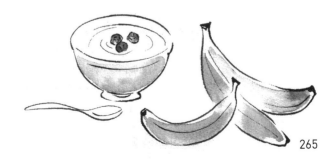

Potato roulade
with beetroot, broccoli
and parsley oil

Serves Four

6 large baking potatoes
4 egg yolks, lightly beaten
4 tbsp potato flour
Rock salt, to taste
Olive oil
2 tbsp sesame seeds

Fresh herbs, such as parsley, basil or
    thyme, finely chopped
3 fresh beetroots, washed and peeled
A pinch of caraway seeds
1 head of broccoli, cut into florettes
4 tbsp olive oil
3 tbsp fresh parsley, chopped

Preheat oven to 170°C, 325°F, gas mark 3.

Bake the potatoes until tender, turning halfway through baking to
prevent browning on the underside. Remove from the oven, and
cool slightly. Cut the potatoes in half, and scrape out the flesh.

Mix this together with the eggs, potato flour, salt and olive oil – in
a food processor, if you like. When it forms a nice stiff dough, use
your hands to knead it; if you find it a bit gluey, add a little more
potato flour.

Grease a 30cm piece of aluminium foil with a little olive oil, and
spread the dough on top. Press with your hands until it is evenly
spread across the foil, about 1cm deep.

Sprinkle with sesame seeds and fresh herbs, and roll it up length-
ways, with the foil pressed around it.

Steam in a steamer, or slowly simmer in a saucepan containing a
little water, for 30 minutes.

While the roulade is cooking, juice one of the beetroots, and chop the remaining two. Boil the chopped beetroot with the juice until tender. Add a pinch of caraway seeds and salt to taste.

Next, gently steam the broccoli florettes in slightly salted water, until tender.

Make the parsley oil by blending together the olive oil and the parsley, in a food processor or liquidiser, until smooth and vibrant green.

Remove the potato roulade from the water, and remove the foil. Cut the roulade into slices about 2cm thick. Arrange the beetroots in the middle of your plate, place a slice of roulade on top, and then scatter the broccoli around. Sprinkle with a few drops of parsley oil, and serve.

Banana mousse

Serves Four

1 banana
50g fresh, soft sheep's or goat's cheese
1 tbsp maple syrup
1 tbsp honey
200ml fresh double cream, whipped
4 fresh mint leaves, to garnish

In a food processor or liquidiser, blend together the banana, cheese, maple syrup and honey, until smooth. Remove from the blender, and carefully fold in the whipped cream.

Decant into four glasses, and garnish each with a fresh mint leaf.

Cream of artichoke base soup

Serves Four

2 fresh globe artichokes
1 litre water

200g potatoes, peeled and chopped
A pinch of rock salt

Boil the artichokes in the water for 20 minutes or until the central leaves will detach with a gentle pull. Remove them from the pan to cool, reserving the cooking water.

Boil the chopped potatoes in the artichoke cooking water until tender.

Pull away the tough outside artichoke leaves and trim the stalk. Put the artichoke hearts and boiled potatoes in a food processor and whizz until very fine. Season with rock salt, reheat and serve.

Mediterranean vegetable spread

Serves Four

Olive oil
150g courgette, chopped
50g aubergine, chopped
40g pitted black olives

60g sheep's yoghurt
150g fresh soft sheep's or goat's cheese
2 tbsp fresh basil
A pinch of rock salt

Heat a few drops of olive oil in a non-stick frying pan and braise the courgette and aubergine for 3–5 minutes until tender. Blend with all remaining ingredients in a food processor until smooth.

Day Thirteen

Porridge *with* fresh fruit and linseed oil

Serves Two

500ml soya, rice or oat milk
50g finely ground oatmeal (or millet, corn or rice flakes)
100g fresh fruit of the season, diced
1 tbsp linseed oil

Heat milk in a small saucepan. Stir in the flakes and boil gently, stirring constantly, for 3 to 5 minutes.

Place the fresh fruit in two bowls, and pour the porridge over top. Sprinkle with linseed oil and serve immediately.

Mixed leaf salad *with* yoghurt dressing

Serves Four

100g live yoghurt (sheep's, goat's, soya or cow's milk)
2 tbsp olive oil
2 tbsp fresh parsley, finely chopped
A pinch of rock salt

500g mixed salad leaves, such as chicory, radicchio and rocket, washed and torn into small pieces
2 tbsp pistachio nuts, finely ground

Pour the yoghurt into a bowl, and add the oil, parsley and salt. Blend together until smooth.

Place the salad leaves on a large plate, and drizzle with the yoghurt dressing. Sprinkle with pistachios, and serve immediately.

Fillet of beef *with* vegetables and potato cubes

Serves Four

200g potatoes
400g beef fillet, cut into 4
A pinch of rock salt
Coconut oil
Fresh rosemary leaves, chopped
100g carrots, chopped
100g courgettes, chopped

100g fennel, chopped
100g broccoli, chopped
100g celery, chopped
125ml water or organic vegetable stock
Fresh herbs, such as basil, rosemary
    and thyme, chopped

Steam or boil the potatoes in their skins in a large pan of water, until tender. When cooled slightly, peel off the skin and cut the potatoes into cubes.

Season the steaks with salt and put to one side. Heat the coconut oil in a frying pan, and quickly fry the steaks, turning frequently, until cooked to taste. Add the potato cubes, and then the chopped rosemary.

In a wok, heat a little more coconut oil, and add the vegetables, stirring constantly. After a few minutes, add the water or stock, cover, and simmer for 2 more minutes, until the vegetables are tender but still crunchy. Remove the lid, and continue simmering until the liquid evaporates.

Serve the steak and potatoes with the vegetables on the side.

Quinoa potato gnocchi *with* fresh spinach, tomatoes and olive cream

Serves Four

550g potatoes, peeled and boiled
4 egg yolks, beaten
3 tbsp potato flour
100g quinoa flour
A pinch of rock salt
A pinch of grated nutmeg

80g Parmesan cheese (plus a little extra to garnish)
500g fresh spinach, washed and stalks removed
1 tsp butter
250g organic baby plum tomatoes
A handful fresh basil leaves, torn

Preheat the oven to 200°C, 400°F, gas mark 6.

Press the potatoes through a sieve or ricer, and blend in a bowl with the egg yolks, potato flour, quinoa flour, salt, nutmeg and Parmesan cheese. Knead together with your hands to form a soft dough.

Quarter the dough, and form 4 rolls, approximately 2cm thick. Cut into pieces, and mould each piece so that it forms a gnocchi. Put to one side to rest.

Place the tomatoes on a baking tray, and roast for about 10 minutes.

To make the olive cream, blend together the pitted black olives and olive oil until smooth. Set to one side.

Fill a saucepan with lightly salted water, and bring to the boil. Simmer the gnocchi for 2 to 3 minutes, and drain.

Next, simmer the spinach in a large covered pot, with only a little water, until tender. Remove the lid, and allow the remaining water to evaporate. Stir in the butter, and a little rock salt and grated nutmeg.

To serve, arrange the gnocchi on a bed of spinach, and gently top with roasted tomatoes. Place a dollop of olive cream on the side, and sprinkle with grated Parmesan and fresh basil leaves. Serve at once.

Day Fourteen

Viva vitality muesli

Serves Two

120g fresh, seasonal fruit, cut into small chunks
120g mixed oat, spelt or millet flakes
50ml cow's, goat's, sheep's or soya milk
10g raisins
30g walnuts, coarsely ground
A few drops of honey

Place the fruit chunks in a bowl, and add the oat flakes (or spelt or millet). Stir in the milk. Sprinkle with raisins and walnuts, and drizzle with honey. Serve at once.

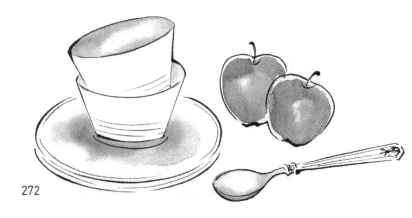

Risotto patties *with* beetroot and asparagus

Serves Four

500g cooked risotto rice	2 cloves
125ml fresh cream	½ tsp ground cinnamon
2 eggs, beaten	1 tsp potato flour
A pinch of rock salt	400g organic asparagus, trimmed
A pinch of grated nutmeg	1 tsp butter
3 tbsp fresh parsley, chopped	Fresh herbs, such as chervil, thyme,
Olive oil	coriander, basil and parsley, finely
1kg beetroot, washed and cubed	chopped, to garnish

In a bowl, blend together the rice, cream, eggs, salt, nutmeg and parsley, and form into small patties or miniature 'burgers'.

Heat a little olive oil in a frying pan, and gently cook the patties, turning frequently, until golden brown.

Next, juice half of the beetroot cubes, and place in a saucepan with the remaining cubes. Add the cloves and cinnamon, and season to taste with a little rock salt. Boil until tender. Dissolve the potato starch in cold water, and stir into the boiling beetroots.

While this is cooking, steam the asparagus until tender, and toss with butter.

To serve, arrange the beetroot on a plate, place the risotto patties on top, and then arrange the asparagus. Sprinkle with fresh herbs, and serve.

Blackberry crème

Serves Four

120g fresh, soft sheep's or goat's cheese
50ml blackberry purée, reserving a little to garnish
2 tbsp honey
250g double cream, whipped
4 fresh mint leaves, to garnish

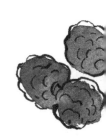

Stir the soft cheese together with the blackberry purée and honey. Fold in the whipped cream.

Spoon into 4 glasses, top with blackberry purée, and garnish with mint leaves.

Potato and lovage soup

Serves Four

1 litre water
A pinch of rock salt
250g potatoes, washed and chopped
A small bunch of fresh lovage, chopped

In a large saucepan, bring the water and salt to the boil, and add the potatoes. Cook until tender.

Cool slightly, and blend in a food processor or liquidiser. When smooth, blend in the lovage. Quickly return to the saucepan and gently reheat. Serve immediately.

Teas and other drinks

On Day Five (see page 85), we looked at some delicious herbal teas, which can be easily prepared at home. Simply add a few teaspoons of dried herbs to some boiling water, cover and leave for a few minutes, and then strain. You may also be able to find some of these herbal teas in teabags, which makes the process even easier! You can flavour your teas with lemon juice, or even a little honey, if desired.

Fresh ginger tea

3–5cm chunk of fresh ginger
Honey, if desired

This requires a little more work, but it has a number of therapeutic benefits (see page 92), as well as being delicious. Slice a good chunk of ginger into thin slices, and put them in a pan with some cold water. You'll need about 5 slices per person. Bring to the boil, take off the heat, and allow the ginger to infuse for about 10 minutes. Reheat, and drink. Add a little honey, if you wish.

Fresh ginger tea drink

50g fresh ginger root
Oranges, sliced
1 tbsp fresh mint leaves, chopped

Bring 1 litre of water to the boil, in a saucepan. Grate 50g fresh ginger root into the water, and turn off the heat. Leave to rest for 5 minutes, and then poor into a jug. Cool and drink with sliced oranges, and freshly chopped mint leaves.

Green tea and lemon verbena

1 tsp green tea
Lemons or limes, sliced

1 tsp fresh lemon verbena leaves, minced
Stevia or honey, if desired

Bring 1 litre of water to the boil, in a saucepan, and add green tea. Let it simmer for about 10 minutes, and then remove from the heat and cool slightly before pouring into a jug. Add some slices of lemon or lime, and freshly minced lemon verbena leaves. To sweeten, add a little stevia (see page 27) or honey. This drink should be enjoyed during the day, as the green tea acts as a stimulant. Don't drink it too late at night.

Cold spiced tea

1 tsp cloves
1 cinnamon stick
1 tsp ground ginger

A pinch of grated nutmeg
Juice of 2 large oranges

Boil up the spices in 1 litre of water and let it steep for 10 minutes. Strain, and leave to cool. Add the orange juice, and a few fresh mint leaves, and serve.

Meadow herb tea

3 tbsp meadow herbs, such as mallow, hibiscus, verbena, mountain everlasting, mint, lemon balm or poppy
Juice of 2 limes, optional

Pour 1 litre of boiling water over the herbs, and steep for 5 minutes. Strain and drink hot, or cool, throughout the day, with lime juice.

Purging tea

½ tbsp yarrow
½ tbsp vermouth (the herb, not the drink made from it)

½ tbsp horsetail
½ tbsp birch leaves
2 stalks lemongrass

Blend together the ingredients, and pour over 1 litre of boiling water. Steep for 2 to 4 minutes, and strain into a jug. Add 2 stalks of crushed lemongrass, and sip warm or cool.

Vegetable broth

This broth is an ideal alkaline drink for in between meals. Ideally, you should aim to drink one or two mugfuls a day, during the 14-day programme.

2 litres cold water
100g celery, sliced
100g carrots, sliced
100g parsnip, sliced

30g potatoes, peeled and sliced
30g mixed herbs, such as basil, marjoram, fennel, parsley, caraway, nutmeg and juniper berries
A pinch of rock salt

Place the cold water in a large cooking pot. Add the vegetables and herbs, as well as a little rock salt. Gently bring to the boil, and then immediately reduce the heat. Simmer for 45 minutes, until the vegetables are tender.

Strain the broth through a sieve, and add a little more rock salt or grated nutmeg to taste. This broth will keep for 2 to 3 days in the fridge.

Alternative Viva Mayr bread

If you don't have time to make the spelt bread, or want a change, why not try this delicious bread, which can be made with either pumpkin or sunflower seeds

Pumpkin seed bread

300g strong wholemeal flour
300g strong white flour
35ml warm water
20g fresh yeast

15g salt
100g pumpkin seed or sunflower seeds
3 tbsp sunflower oil

Using a mixer with a dough hook, blend together the flours, water, yeast and salt. Continue 'kneading' for 10 minutes. Leave to rest for 30 minutes, and then knead again.

Cut the two into small pieces, to create little rolls, of approximately 50g each.

Place the rolls on a slightly floured baking tray, brush with water, and sprinkle with pumpkin seeds or sunflower seeds. Cover with aluminium foil, and leave to rest for 20 minutes.

Preheat the oven to 180°C, 350°F, gas mark 4.

Bake the rolls for 12 to 14 minutes.

Viva Mayr spreads

Each of these serves four, and can be substituted for any of the spreads suggested in the daily menus.

Herbal spread

200g fresh, unsalted soft goat's or sheep's cheese
50g mixed fresh herbs, such as chervil, parsley, basil, coriander, sage or tarragon, chopped
2–3 tbsp cold-pressed extra-virgin olive oil
A pinch of rock salt

Blend all of the ingredients together in a food processor or liquidiser, until smooth and creamy.

Fresh trout spread

200g smoked trout fillets
100g fresh, soft sheep's or goat's cheese
100g potatoes, cooked and pressed through a sieve
1 tsp fresh horseradish
1 tsp fresh dill, finely chopped
A pinch of rock salt

Blend all of the ingredients together in a food processor or liquidiser, until smooth and creamy.

Mediterranean vegetable spread

1 tsp olive oil
150g courgettes, chopped
50 g aubergine, chopped
40g pitted black olives

60g live yoghurt (sheep's or goat's)
150g fresh, soft sheep's or goat's cheese
2 tbsp fresh basil, chopped
A pinch of rock salt

Heat the olive oil in a frying pan, and cook the courgettes and aubergines until tender, stirring frequently (about 3 to 5 minutes). Remove from the heat, and tip into a food processor or liquidiser, along with all of the remaining ingredients. Whizz until smooth.

Avocado spread

2 ripe and soft avocados, peeled
   and stoned
Juice of half a lime
200g fresh, soft sheep's or goat's cheese

1 tsp basil, finely chopped
1 tbsp sesame seeds
A pinch of rock salt

Blend together all of the ingredients in a food processor or liquidiser until smooth. Season to taste, and then serve.

Vitamin spread

200g carrots, chopped
200g celery, chopped
200g broccoli, chopped
150g potatoes, chopped (you may
   substitute hemp or soya tofu, if desired)

3 tsp hemp oil (or linseed oil)
2 tbsp blend of chervil, basil
   and parsley, finely chopped
A pinch of rock salt

Place the carrots, celery, broccoli and potatoes in a saucepan with a little water or organic stock. Cook until tender. Drain, and then tip into a food processor or liquidiser with the remaining ingredients. Whizz until smooth.

Pumpkin spread

100g fresh pumpkin, peeled, fibres removed, and chopped
350g fresh, soft sheep's or goat's cheese
50g pumpkin seeds, finely ground
3 tbsp cold-pressed pumpkin-seed oil

In a large saucepan, simmer the pumpkin in enough water to cover, for about 3 to 4 minutes, or until tender. Tip into a food processor or liquidiser with the remaining ingredients. Whizz until smooth.

Potato and tofu spread

200g fresh silken tofu
200g potatoes, boiled and skins removed
2 tbsp soya oil (or hemp or linseed oil)
A pinch of rock salt
A pinch of grated nutmeg

Press the potatoes through a ricer, and blend in a food processor or liquidiser with the remaining ingredients. Whizz until smooth, and serve immediately.

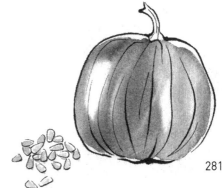

Useful Contacts

The Viva Centre for Modern Mayr Medicine is situated in Maria Wörth, a small village on the banks of the Wörthersee, an alpine lake near Klagenfurt in southern Austria. It is set within a luxurious 5-star hotel.

The Viva Centre
Das Zentrum für Moderne Mayr Medizin
Seepromenade 11
A-9082 Maria Wörth
Austria

For information, tel: 00 43 42 73 31117

Website: www.viva-mayr.com
Email enquiries: office@viva-mayr.com

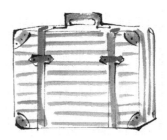

17584562R00171

Printed in Poland
by Amazon Fulfillment
Poland Sp. z o.o., Wrocław